NURSING AND HEALTH CARE

EDITOR: LYNNE WIGENS AND JANE DAY

MENTORSHIP AND CLINICAL SUPERVISION SKILLS IN HEALTH CARE

SECOND EDITION

Lynne Wigens and Rachel Heathershaw

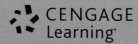

CENGAGE
Learning

Australia • Brazil • Canada • Mexico • Singapore • Spain • United Kingdom • United States

CENGAGE
Learning

**Mentorship and Clinical Supervision Skills
in Health Care, Second Edition**
Lynne Wigens and Rachel Heathershaw

Publishing Director: Linden Harris

Commissioning Editor: Annabel Ainscow

Production Editor: Beverley Copland

Production Controller: Eyvett Davis

Marketing Manager: Lauren Mottram

Typesetter: Integra Software Services
Pvt. Ltd.

Cover design: Adam Renvoize

For product information and technology assistance,
contact **emea.info@cengage.com.**
For permission to use material from this text or product,
and for permission queries,
email **emea.permissions@cengage.com.**

British Library Cataloguing-in-Publication Data
A catalogue record for this book is available from the British Library.

ISBN: 978-1-4080-7506-7

Cengage Learning EMEA
Cheriton House, North Way, Andover, Hampshire, SP10 5BE,
United Kingdom

Cengage Learning products are represented in Canada by Nelson
Education Ltd.

For your lifelong learning solutions, visit **www.cengage.co.uk**

Purchase your next print book, e-book or e-chapter at
www.cengagebrain.com

Printed in China by RR Donnelley
1 2 3 4 5 6 7 8 9 10 – 15 14 13

CONTENTS

PREFACE

Health care professionals learn constantly through their practice. This second edition of *Mentorship and Clinical Supervision Skills in Health Care* continues to aim to provide newly qualified health professionals, mentors and students with the background, theory and practical knowledge to get the most out of practice and to harness all forms of learning opportunity. It also seeks to remind practitioners that the skills required to support learning have common themes, which are transferable, regardless of the professional discipline you belong to. Our interest in learning through practice is based on many years of working and teaching within education and service settings, as senior lecturers and senior nurses. The book is also in line with the current vision and strategy of Jane Cummings, Chief Nursing Officer for England, that Nurses, Midwives and Care-Givers should have the following 'Six Cs' values to unite their professions: care; compassion; competence; communication; courage and commitment.

The book is divided into chapters covering key areas. In each chapter the subject is considered from the stance of a student as well as that of a qualified health care professional (mentors, practice teachers, preceptors, clinical supervisors and practice educators), using theoretical and practical examples.

What makes this book different from many other texts is that it looks at individual and social learning, which, we believe, are inextricably linked. The book is, therefore, context related, focuses on the practical appreciation of learning theories, and covers the principles of sound mentorship and clinical supervision. This book incorporates evidence regarding situated learning, an awareness of the key drivers in practice learning currently, and the influence of learning communities on the health care practice of students and qualified staff. It also suggests the components that come together to make a 'good' clinical learning environment. Whether you are a student or an experienced practitioner, this book should offer insights to improve your own learning and your contribution to the learning of others. We hope it may even be transformative in the way that you think about practice-based learning. Moon (2004) reminds us that as teachers we can only hope that a student learns. According to her, teaching can occur in a different place to the learning and learning can happen without teaching. However teaching without the learner as the focus is pointless.

ACKNOWLEDGEMENTS

As co-authors of this book we would like to thank the health professional colleagues, educationalists, students and patients who have influenced the thinking that informs this text.

We also should take the opportunity to personally thank our families for their unfaltering support, especially Paul, Matt and Sam Wigens and Tanne and Kit Heathershaw.

We are reminded in developing this second edition that:

'You cannot step into the same river twice. Not only is the context constantly changing, you also continually transform as you act and learn.'

Heraclitus, Greek Philosopher

The publishers would like to thank Helen Ashwood, Mike Parkinson and Ben Stanfield-Davies for their insightful review comments on the manuscript.

ABOUT THE AUTHORS

Dr Lynne Wigens Lynne is currently Director of Nursing and Quality at the Ipswich Hospital NHS Trust, and was previously Director of Patient Safety and Clinical Quality for Suffolk. She is the author of the first edition of this book. Lynne has written journal articles on a range of topics including; critical care, lay caring, change strategies, learning through practice, expert and multidisciplinary care, human resource management and recruitment. Throughout her career Lynne has worked in senior clinical, education and management roles at both regional and national level. A key motivation throughout her career has been to ensure that healthcare practice is the best it can be through improving services in a range of ways. Lynne has been a Nursing and Midwifery Council Reviewer, Member of the Royal College of Nursing Eastern Region Board and is currently a Visiting Senior Fellow in Nursing at University Campus Suffolk.

Rachel Heathershaw Rachel is currently Senior Lecturer in Practice Learning and Development at University Campus Suffolk, in Ipswich. Rachel's main teaching responsibilities centre on Preparation for Mentorship and Leadership and Service Innovation. She leads the delivery of the MA Leadership and Service Innovation course and teaches on leadership, management and communication across foundation degrees, pre- and post-registration, and post-graduate courses. Rachel's interests are exploring evaluation of placement experience, and developing learning in practice and mentorship from a variety of health care perspectives.

During her nursing career, Rachel worked predominantly in acute medicine and rehabilitation, as a ward manager and staff nurse. She then moved to the role of Clinical Practice Facilitator supporting practice learning. This role developed further to encompass a broader educational perspective, including the coordination and organization of a range of clinical education programmes and specific project work. During this time Rachel studied for a BSc Hons degree in Nursing Practice at Suffolk College and an MA in Leadership and Innovation in Health and Social Care.

Series Editors for the *Nursing and Health Care Practice* Series:

Dr Lynne Wigens, Director of Nursing and Quality at The Ipswich Hospital NHS Trust. Visiting Senior Fellow University Campus Suffolk

Dr Jane Day, Head of Division, Practice Learning and Midwifery, School of Nursing and Midwifery, University Campus Suffolk

WALK THROUGH TOUR

CHAPTER 2

LEARNING FROM AND IN CLINICAL PRACTICE

LEARNING OBJECTIVES

By the end of this chapter you should be able to:

- explain adult and higher education perspectives on learning
- appreciate the differences between behaviourist, cognitive and humanistic theories of learning
- understand the importance of lifelong learning and continuous professional development to professional practice
- understand your increasing involvement as a team member in the clinical environment
- anticipate the challenges of entering different communities of practice and how this impacts on your professional identity.

INTRODUCTION

In this chapter you will explore educational theories to aid understanding of learning through practice. We will consider a range of theories of learning broadly termed behaviourist, cognitive and humanistic and look at the importance of these and their impact on learning in health care environments. Some educational issues are common to all professions such as adult and higher education perspectives on learning. In other ways, however, the health care setting is special in the way that this impacts on individual and collective learning. We will be thinking about the clinical teams and about situated learning in clinical environments. You will explore the relationship between participating in clinical practice and the social environment and learning.

5

Learning objectives: Listed at the beginning of each chapter, these emphasize the key topics that need to be understood before progressing to the next chapter.

---

person holistically as they grow and develop throughout their life. Feedback about learning is internal to the 'self' and based on individual motivations, goal setting and areas of interest. As learning is understood to be subjective, individual and based on experience, this way of looking at learning can alternatively be called *phenomenological*. Learning has its ultimate goal *self-actualization*, not just behavioural change but changes in values, attitudes and beliefs.

Humanism is often linked to the adult education movement and the concept of andragogy. Andragogy has been defined as the 'art and science' of helping adults to learn. The term 'lifelong learning' (discussed in more detail on p. 19) rejects the model of education that is confined to childhood and early adulthood. Andragogy is based on six main assumptions (Knowles, 1990):

1 Adults need to know *why* they need to learn something.
2 Adults have a self-concept where they are responsible for their decisions and need to be treated in a way that acknowledges this self-direction.
3 Adult learners bring a wealth of previous experience to their current learning.
4 Adults are ready to learn something that has relevance to their everyday life.
5 Adults tend to be 'problem centred' in their learning.
6 Motivation mainly comes from 'internal' pressures, e.g. increased job satisfaction, self-esteem, and quality of life.

Knowles (1990) views an adult learner as having the following characteristics. They:

- respond best to a non-threatening learning environment where there is a good teacher–learner relationship
- want to assess themselves against a relevant standard to determine educational needs
- want to select their own learning experiences – self-directing
- prefer a problem-orientated, patient-based approach to learning
- want to apply their knowledge and skills immediately
- want to know how they are progressing
- want to contribute from their own knowledge and skills to help others to learn.

Although this view of adult learners still has some relevance it has been much criticized, particularly for the implied absence of self-directed and problem-based learning from the area of children's learning (Tennant, 2005). There is still a need to view adults as actively engaged in continuing education over time and in a range of settings and to see learning through continuous education as integral to all the roles that people undertake

Phenomenological Phenomenology takes the intuitive experience of phenomena (what presents itself to us in conscious experience) as its starting point and tries to extract from it the essential features of experiences and the holistic essence of what we experience

Self-actualization An individual is able to fully use and express their talents, capabilities and potential

Key word definitions: These are succinct definitions in the margin for important terms that are highlighted in the text.

---

are 'instrumental conditioning' (Thorndike, 1913) and 'operant conditioning' (Skinner, 1953).

An environmental event (e.g. a patient having a cardiac arrest) may act as a stimulus, and the outcome of the individual's response to the stimulus can be either negative or positive. An example of a positive outcome to this environmental situation could be that the student found they were able to respond quickly to deliver basic life support even though they had not undertaken this in practice before. A possible negative outcome could be when a student responds by freezing and moving away from the patient, not instituting basic life support.

Reinforcement will lead to a change in behaviour, either to increase or decrease the likelihood of the behaviour recurring. In the previous example of a positive outcome from the student's response to a stimulus, the student is likely to develop increased confidence in their basic life support skills. Rewards such as feeling more confident in their practice or being praised by the mentor are examples of 'reinforcers' for a desired behaviour.

Reflective activity

Being asked to carry out 'basic' care whilst an opportunity to develop clinical skills is missed could be regarded as a negative outcome and loss of a range of behaviours. Think about what behaviours the student might increase or decrease as a result of this negative situation, and what further actions this could lead to.

Behaviourist learning focuses on observable behaviours that occur as a result of consequences or beliefs and achieving goals or objectives, so you can see why many educators view learning in this way. The development of pre-specified objectives for educational experiences is based on behaviourist theories of learning and these are the basis for reliable and valid educational planning and assessment. The central contention is that educational goals should be specified beforehand and the way to assess learning should also be expressed in terms of observable and measurable behaviour. The arguments for pre-specifying objectives to direct and measure learning are powerful; however, there are objections. A behaviourist view of human beings, learning and the nature of knowledge can be seen as manipulative and as taking focus away from the personal, active, individual aspects of learning which can be intrinsically valuable. Table 2.1 includes the names of some theorists who have investigated this approach to learning. Behaviourism has been much criticized, even after recent revisions, for falling short in its understanding of human personalities and different responses. It is difficult for this approach to learning to explain why some people continue to display negative behavioural responses.

Reflective activity: An opportunity to undertake structured reflection on the topics under discussion.

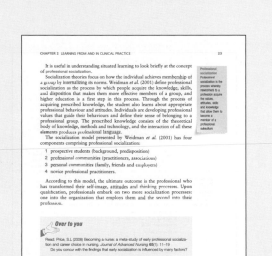

It is useful in understanding situated learning to look briefly at the concept of professional socialization.

Socialization theories focus on how the individual achieves membership of a group by internalizing its norms. Weidman *et al.* (2001) define professional socialization as the process by which people acquire the knowledge, skills, and disposition that makes them more effective members of a group, and higher education is a first step in this process. Through the process of acquiring prescribed knowledge, the student also learns about appropriate professional behaviour and attitudes. Individuals are developing professional values that guide their behaviours and define their sense of belonging to a professional group. The prescribed knowledge consists of the theoretical body of knowledge, methods and technology, and the interaction of all these elements produce professional language.

The socialization model presented by Weidman *et al.* (2001) has four components comprising professional socialization:

1 prospective students (background, predisposition)
2 professional communities (practitioners, associations)
3 personal communities (family, friends and employers)
4 novice professional practitioners.

According to this model, the ultimate outcome is the professional who has transformed their self-image, attitudes and thinking processes. Upon qualification, professionals embark on two more socialization processes: one into the organization that employs them and the second into their profession.

Over to you

Read: Price, S.L (2008) Becoming a nurse: a meta-study of early professional socialization and career choice in nursing. *Journal of Advanced Nursing* 65(1): 11–19
Do you concur with the findings that early socialization is influenced by many factors?

Although professional socialization is an aspect of situated learning, Wenger (1998) suggests that education needs to be understood as changing identity in a lifelong process, not merely in terms of an initial period of socialization into a subculture, such as a profession. Learning through practice becomes a mutual development process between individuals and communities. There is a subtle difference between the imitation and internalization of norms and the construction of identities within communities of practice.

Professional socialization Professional socialization is the process whereby newcomers to a profession acquire the values, attitudes, skills and knowledge that allow them to become a member of a professional subculture

Over to you: This feature encourages you to find out more about or follow up on the issues raised in the text.

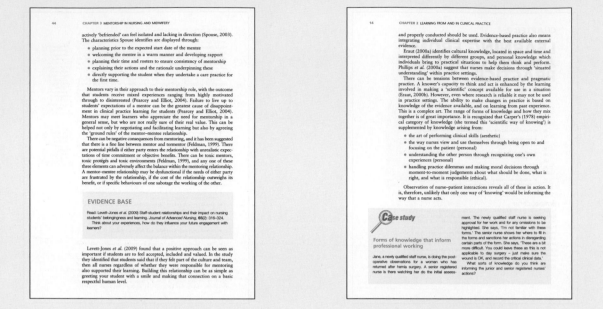

Evidence base: This provides well-founded evidence-based research about the topic for you to read.

Case study: These scenarios are drawn from multi-professional settings to demonstrate learning points and encourage you to think about how you practise and learn.

Health care professional speaks: A range of health care professionals talk about practical situations and caseload management issues (fictitious).

Student speaks: Students, from a range of health care professions, talk about their experiences of various situations (fictitious).

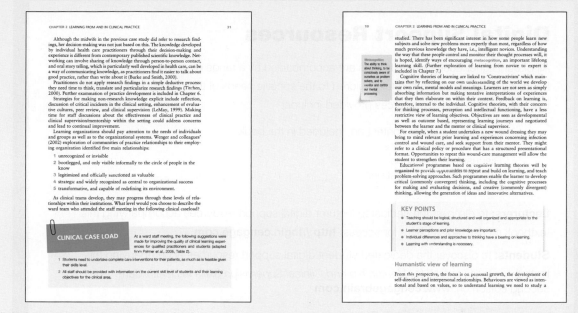

Clinical case load: Demonstrate the link between theory and practice by discussing how issues are dealt with in the workplace.

Key points: Summarize the main points in the preceding text.

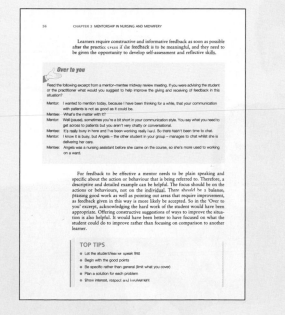

Top tips: Provide tips for best practice.

Rapid recap: At the end of each chapter, these give the reader a chance to assess what they have learnt from reading the text. Answers are provided in the appendix.

Digital Support Resources

All of our Higher Education textbooks are accompanied by a range of digital support resources. Each title's resources are carefully tailored to the specific needs of the particular book's readers. Examples of the kind of resources provided include:

- Additional chapter content not included in the book
- Self-test quiz questions
- Discussion Questions
- Critical Thinking Questions
- PowerPoint slides

Lecturers: to discover the dedicated lecturer digital support resources accompanying this textbook please register here for access: **http://login.cengage.com**.

Students: to discover the dedicated student digital support resources accompanying this textbook, please search for *Mentorship and Clinical Supervision Skills in Health Care* second edition on: **www.cengagebrain.com**

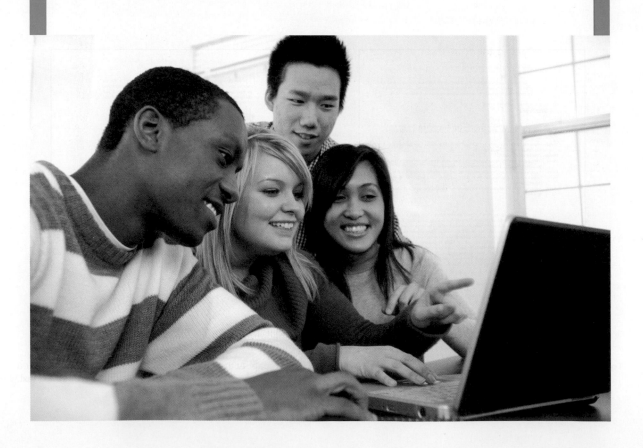

CHAPTER 1
MENTORSHIP AND CLINICAL SUPERVISION SKILLS – AN INTRODUCTION

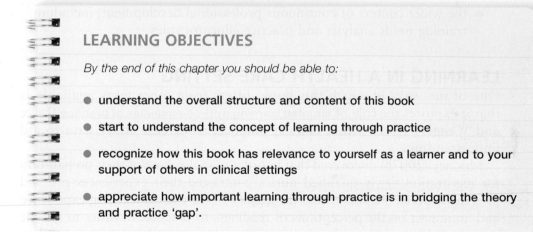

LEARNING OBJECTIVES

By the end of this chapter you should be able to:

- understand the overall structure and content of this book

- start to understand the concept of learning through practice

- recognize how this book has relevance to yourself as a learner and to your support of others in clinical settings

- appreciate how important learning through practice is in bridging the theory and practice 'gap'.

INTRODUCTION

In this book you will examine learning through practice, what it is and why it is important, not only for your own learning and for the development of your professional practice, but also for supporting others in their clinical learning. The purpose of this introductory chapter is to set the scene. You can then approach the rest of the book with an understanding of what you are trying to achieve in developing your learning from your practice experiences. We have also used this section to introduce the rest of the book to you.

The book covers a range of issues, theories and practical examples regarding learning through practice and is a helpful resource for students who want to get the most from their clinical placements and for mentors and supervisors who facilitate learning within clinical settings. Using evidence and research throughout, the book demonstrates the practical application of situated learning and learning communities within health care education and offers a range of interactive exercises and case studies.

The following aspects of learning through practice are examined:

- making the best of use of clinical learning opportunities
- identifying individual learning needs, i.e. learning contracts and personal development plans
- clinical supervision, mentorship and preceptorship
- problem-based and action learning
- evidencing practice learning, i.e. portfolios, competencies, assessment and evaluation facilitation of learning
- the adult learner and lifelong learning
- improving the learning environment and managing constraints
- the wider context of continuous professional development, including training needs analysis and practice educator roles.

Situated learning
Situated learning takes place in the setting where the learning will be applied, and assumes that social processes will affect this learning

Communities of practice
Learning is seen as an act of membership and participation in a community of practice, which is the social group that integrates knowledge and situated learning into its life and working

LEARNING IN A HEALTH CARE SETTING

One of the ways in which this book differs from other texts available is that it explores the role of situated learning and communities of practice (Lave and Wenger, 1991) within clinical practice, using case study data to aid understanding.

Mooney (2007b) discovered that in order to make sense of their preparation for registration newly qualified nurses contrasted their experiences pre and post registration. She found that the quality of the clinical learning experience had an impact on the perceptions of readiness to practice. In order to get the most from learning through practice it is necessary to appreciate the complexity of learning within a health care setting. Take a look at the following case study, in which a registered nurse is observed going about her work on a hospital ward.

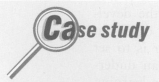

Case study

Prioritizing work in a practice setting

A nurse was walking at a fast pace to get behind the nurses' station. During the first ten minutes on the ward, I observed that she made decisions about the following:

1 She decided to telephone the police because a patient had died and she had been unable to contact the next of kin; she made the call.

2 She listened to a doctor's request for her to take out a cannula from a patient, as this was no longer in the right place (extravasation or

tissued), and to do a sitting and standing blood pressure recording to look for postural hypotension with another patient. Although acknowledging the request, she did not fulfil it during the ten-minute period.

3 She spoke in a welcoming way to a patient, who was being transferred on his bed from the High Dependency Unit (HDU), following bowel surgery. The nurse noted that the patient's documentation was not suitable for this particular ward and so she took a few core care plans over to the patient and said, 'I'll catch up on the paperwork later'.

4 She walked around to a whiteboard that had all the patients' names on it and said to the student nurse working with her, 'Some of this care can be done this afternoon, because we won't have time this morning – like the removal of the epidural and the CVP (central venous pressure) line on the HDU transfer'.

How do you think this registered nurse had learnt to set priorities for the work that she had to do during the ten-minute period of the observation?

From reading this observational account, it starts to become clear that health care practitioners have to learn to meet many requirements at the same time. Indeed, the greatest nursing competence could be the ability to manage multiple demands. The nurse in the case study may have been surprised if you had asked her how she 'learnt' to deal with these demands, but one thing is pretty certain: she is unlikely to say that this was how she was taught during her nursing education. A student practitioner watching a qualified member of staff may find it difficult to grasp the 'knowledge' that underpins their work, particularly as every interpretation involves a point of view. As a practitioner goes about their professional work, their use of knowledge and their own knowledge creation cannot easily be separated because the use of an idea in a new context is itself a minor act of knowledge creation.

Health care practitioners perceive, experience, and learn to manage everyday practice in contexts where many things happen at the same time. As the record of the short observation given in the previous case study illustrates, it would be impractical to halt nursing practice to examine critically the processes in which nurses engage and through which they are learning to manage practice. Johns (2006) suggests that learning as a result of reflection is both deliberative and intuitive and can occur within or after practice. Paradoxically, as the observational excerpt shows, time for such reflection in practice is constrained by the need to act 'now', and a nurse soon develops a foundation of tacit knowledge to use in her daily tasks. Consequently, practice learning remains largely implicit, and part of the task of this book is to help you to engage with and get the most from your practice and that of others.

Tacit knowledge
This is the knowledge that people carry in their minds that they have learned from their experience, which they may not be aware of. It is seen as valuable to others as it is rooted in context, people, places, ideas and experiences. (Polanyi (1951) originated this concept).

USING THIS BOOK

In this book, we wish to reinforce the approach that learning is not a passive exercise and that the most effective way to learn from the written material is for you to interact with what you are reading. This is accomplished in a number of ways, particularly by considering the text in the light of your own experiences.

Each chapter commences by identifying the key elements that you will learn about in the text and contains activities that illustrate the issues with which the chapter deals. Through engagement with these activities you will see how the ideas presented translate into your own and other people's experiences. One example of this will be a 'reflective activity' that gives you time to reflect on the ideas that you are meeting and relate them in some way to your own experiences. As a result, you will be acquiring and consolidating the skills for learning through practice as you progress through the book. Throughout the book, you will meet new terms, ideas and words, which will be identified and explained. So that the use of educational terminology does not impede understanding, 'key words' will be defined in the margin, to help you to 'translate' the words for your own use and become comfortable with using the words and the concepts that they incorporate. A few 'rapid recap' questions are offered at the end of each chapter to allow you an opportunity to examine 'what you have learnt'.

The overall content of this book looks at learning as being both socially based and individualistic.

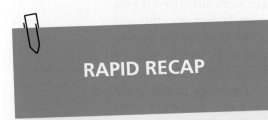

RAPID RECAP

Check your progress so far by working through each of the following questions.

1 What is situated learning?

2 What is a community of practice?

3 Define the term 'tacit knowledge'

4 Give some examples of evidence that could be used within a professional portfolio.

If you have difficulty with any of these questions, read through the section again to refresh your understanding before moving on.

CHAPTER 2

LEARNING FROM AND IN CLINICAL PRACTICE

LEARNING OBJECTIVES

By the end of this chapter you should be able to:

- explain adult and higher education perspectives on learning

- appreciate the differences between behaviourist, cognitive and humanistic theories of learning

- understand the importance of lifelong learning and continuous professional development to professional practice

- understand your increasing involvement as a team member in the clinical environment

- anticipate the challenges of entering different communities of practice and how this impacts on your professional identity.

Bonus features for this chapter available on the book's website

INTRODUCTION

In this chapter you will explore educational theories to aid understanding of learning through practice. We will consider a range of theories of learning broadly termed behaviourist, cognitive and humanistic and look at the importance of these and their impact on learning in health care environments. Some educational issues are common to all professions such as adult and higher education perspectives on learning. In other ways, however, the health care setting is special in the way that this impacts on individual and collective learning. We will be thinking about the clinical teams and about situated learning in clinical environments. You will explore the relationship between participating in clinical practice and the social environment and learning.

EDUCATION THEORIES FOR PRACTICE

Learning is something everyone does all of the time. There are two main stances on learning and the process of learning. It can be seen as either:

1 **Outcome based** – knowledge is taken in and absorbed by the learner and retained for future use; this is a building block approach, where knowledge is accumulated. Gagné (1985) took a systems view of learning, seeing information as being processed. The key elements involved in a systems way of looking at learning are the learner, the stimulus situation, the learner's memory, and their response to the situation. What is learnt may include intellectual skills, information, cognitive strategies, psychomotor skills, or attitudes.

> ❝ *Learning is a change in human disposition or capability that persists over a period of time and is not simply ascribable to the process of growth.*
>
> *Gagné, 1985, p. 2*

2 **Process based** – this entails a flexible network of ideas, knowledge and feelings, where learning involves a process of assembling, ordering or modifying understanding (termed 'assimilation' by Piaget, 1971). Learning as a process is grounded in experience, requiring resolution of conflicts between alternative ways of looking at and adapting to the world. It involves transactions between the learner and the environment and leads to the creation of knowledge.

> ❝ *Learning is the process whereby knowledge is created through the transformation of experience.*
>
> *Kolb, 1984a, p. 38*

The student's conception of what learning is, either as a product, a process, or both, can predict the quality of their learning (Marton and Saljo, 1984). The way that a learner views their learning affects whether learning is at a surface level or a deep level. It has been suggested that there are five main levels, with levels 1 to 3 perceived as 'surface' and levels 4 and 5 as 'deep' (Marton and Saljo, 1984).

Levels of learning

1 Learning is about increasing knowledge
2 Learning is about memorizing and remembering
3 Learning is acquiring facts or skills to be used
4 Learning is about making sense and determining the meaning
5 Learning is about understanding reality

Learning that is deep and process based has perhaps been more influential within many professional education programmes. More recently, there has also been a movement to combine process and product within theories of learning. For instance, Jarvis (1995) combined both in the following 'meanings of learning':

- any more or less permanent change in behaviour which occurs as a result of practice
- a relatively permanent behavioural change as a result of experience
- the process whereby knowledge is created through the transformation of experience
- the process of transforming experience to knowledge, skills and attitudes
- memorizing information.

Whether learning is meaningful is dependent on the learner's relationship to this new knowledge and their current cognitive working (Pardoe, 2000). For this interpretation of learning to help resolve the outcome versus process debate, it is crucial to read Jarvis's (1995) meanings of learning from a stance that assumes that the terms 'experience' and 'practice' do not just refer to an individual but to the wider social context.

As well as understanding that individual factors affect learning, it is important to appreciate that the meaning of learning is not determined alone, but in conjunction with the experience of others in a socially and culturally agreed form (Lave and Wenger, 1991).

PERSPECTIVES ON LEARNING

Apart from the outcome and process ways, there are three main psychological approaches to understanding learning. In this section of the chapter, you will explore the behaviourist, cognitive and humanistic perspectives on learning and see how these may influence mentors and clinical supervisors in clinical settings.

Behaviourist learning theory

From a behaviourist stance, learning is the result of the application of consequences, that is, learners begin to connect certain responses with certain stimuli. According to behaviourism, there are two components to learning – Stimulus>Response. Different behavioural theories elaborate on this basic paradigm in different ways. Within the classical conditioning model, learning starts with an unconditioned response (a reflex) to an unconditioned (positive or negative) stimulus.

Other models focus on the consequence of the action, whether pleasant or otherwise. This adds another component to learning – Stimulus>Response>Outcome. Examples of theories that look at learning in this way are 'instrumental conditioning' (Thorndike, 1913) and 'operant conditioning' (Skinner, 1953).

An environmental event (e.g. a patient having a cardiac arrest) may act as a stimulus, and the outcome of the individual's response to the stimulus can be either negative or positive. An example of a positive outcome to this environmental situation could be that the student found they were able to respond quickly to deliver basic life support even though they had not undertaken this in practice before. A possible negative outcome could be when a student responds by freezing and moving away from the patient, not instituting basic life support.

Reinforcement will lead to a change in behaviour, either to increase or decrease the likelihood of the behaviour recurring. In the previous example of a positive outcome from the student's response to a stimulus, the student is likely to develop increased confidence in their basic life support skills. Rewards such as feeling more confident in their practice or being praised by the mentor are examples of 'reinforcers' for a desired behaviour.

Reflective activity

Being asked to carry out 'basic' care whilst an opportunity to develop clinical skills is missed could be regarded as a negative outcome and lead to a range of behaviours. Think about what behaviours the student might increase or decrease as a result of this negative situation, and what further actions this could lead to.

Behaviourist learning focuses on observable behaviours that occur as a result of consequences or beliefs and achieving goals or objectives, so you can see why many educators view learning in this way. The development of pre-specified objectives for educational experiences is based on behaviourist theories of learning and these are the basis for reliable and valid educational planning and assessment. The central contention is that educational goals should be specified beforehand and the way to assess learning should also be expressed in terms of observable and measurable behaviour. The arguments for pre-specifying objectives to direct and measure learning are powerful; however, there are objections. A behaviourist view of human beings, learning and the nature of knowledge can be seen as manipulative and as taking focus away from the personal, active, individual aspects of learning which can be intrinsically valuable.

Table 2.1 includes the names of some theorists who have investigated this approach to learning. Behaviourism has been much criticized, even after recent revisions, for falling short in its understanding of human personalities and different responses. It is difficult for this approach to learning to explain why some people continue to display negative behavioural responses.

Educational programmes based on behaviourist views of learning might be competence based and promote standardization of practice.

Table 2.1 Learning theories, theorists and the role of the mentor/clinical supervisor

Theory	Behaviourist	Cognitive	Humanistic
Theorists	Skinner Thorndike Watson	Bruner Gagné Piaget	Knowles Maslow Rogers
Role of the mentor	Learning outcome setter Behaviour modifier	Role model Disseminator of information Prompter	Facilitator Coach Listener

Reflective activity

Do you identify individual, personal objectives for learning in practice, or do you concentrate only on learning objectives defined by the educational programme for placement learning?

KEY POINTS

- Activity is important
- Frequent practice and repetition help in generalizing and discriminating
- Reinforcement is the main motivating force
- Learning is helped by clear objectives

Cognitive theory

Cognitive theorists view learning as coming from experience, reasoning and the remembering of information that allows a person to adapt to the environment. Learning is about knowing, discovering and making meaning through intellectual processing and mental structuring. Understanding learning requires the study of information processing, as learning requires varying levels of elaboration moving from perception to the making of meaning. Remembering can be enhanced when, through experience, a person adds more connections to a single concept.

The cognitive processes that are the basis of the differing developmental stages between infancy and adulthood and from novice to expert have been studied. There has been significant interest in how some people learn new subjects and solve new problems more expertly than most, regardless of how much previous knowledge they have, i.e., intelligent novices. Understanding the way that these people control and monitor their thought processes will, it is hoped, identify ways of encouraging metacognition, an important lifelong learning skill. (Further exploration of learning from novice to expert is included in Chapter 7.)

Metacognition
The ability to think about thinking, to be consciously aware of ourselves as problem solvers, and to monitor and control our mental processing

Cognitive theories of learning are linked to 'Constructivism' which maintains that by reflecting on our own understanding of the world we develop our own rules, mental models and meanings. Learners are not seen as simply absorbing information but making tentative interpretations of experiences that they then elaborate on within their context. Feedback on learning is, therefore, internal to the individual. Cognitive theorists, with their concern for thinking processes, perception and intellectual functioning, have a less restrictive view of learning objectives. Objectives are seen as developmental as well as outcome based, representing learning journeys and negotiated between the learner and the mentor or clinical supervisor.

For example, when a student undertakes a new wound dressing they may bring to mind relevant prior learning and experiences concerning infection control and wound care, and seek support from their mentor. They might refer to a clinical policy or procedure that has a structured presentational format. Opportunities to repeat this wound-care management will allow the student to strengthen their learning.

Educational programmes based on cognitive learning theories will be organized to provide opportunities to repeat and build on learning, and teach problem-solving approaches. Such programmes enable the learner to develop critical (commonly convergent) thinking, including the cognitive processes for making and evaluating decisions, and creative (commonly divergent) thinking, allowing the generation of ideas and innovative alternatives.

KEY POINTS

- Teaching should be logical, structured and well organized and appropriate to the student's stage of learning.
- Learner perceptions and prior knowledge are important.
- Individual differences and approaches to thinking have a bearing on learning.
- Learning *with* understanding is necessary.

Humanistic view of learning

From this perspective, the focus is on personal growth, the development of self-direction and interpersonal relationships. Behaviours are viewed as intentional and based on values, so to understand learning we need to study a person holistically as they grow and develop throughout their life. Feedback about learning is internal to the 'self' and based on individual motivations, goal setting and areas of interest. As learning is understood to be subjective, individual and based on experience, this way of looking at learning can alternatively be called phenomenogical. Learning has as its ultimate goal self-actualization, not just behavioural change but changes in values, attitudes and beliefs.

Humanism is often linked to the adult education movement and the concept of andragogy. Andragogy has been defined as the 'art and science' of helping adults to learn. The term 'lifelong learning' (discussed in more detail on p. 15) rejects the model of education that is confined to childhood and early adulthood. Andragogy is based on six main assumptions (Knowles, 1990):

1 Adults need to know *why* they need to learn something.

2 Adults have a self-concept where they are responsible for their decisions and need to be treated in a way that acknowledges this self-direction.

3 Adult learners bring a wealth of previous experience to their current learning.

4 Adults are ready to learn something that has relevance to their everyday life.

5 Adults tend to be 'problem centred' in their learning.

6 Motivation mainly comes from 'internal' pressures, e.g. increased job satisfaction, self-esteem, and quality of life.

Knowles (1990) views an adult learner as having the following characteristics. They:

● respond best to a non-threatening learning environment where there is a good teacher–learner relationship

● want to assess themselves against a relevant standard to determine educational needs

● want to select their own learning experiences – self-directing

● prefer a problem-orientated, patient-based approach to learning

● want to apply their knowledge and skills immediately

● want to know how they are progressing

● want to contribute from their own knowledge and skills to help others to learn.

Although this view of adult learners still has some relevance it has been much criticized, particularly for the implied absence of self-directed and problem-based learning from the area of children's learning (Tennant, 2005). There is still a need to view adults as actively engaged in continuing education over time and in a range of settings and to see learning through continuous education as integral to all the roles that people undertake

Phenomenogical
Phenomenology takes the intuitive experience of phenomena (what presents itself to us in conscious experience) as its starting point and tries to extract from it the essential features of experiences and the holistic essence of what we experience

Self-actualization
An individual is able to fully use and express their talents, capabilities and potential

throughout their life. Education and learning is about dialogue, about giving the student the space and support to develop their ideas and themselves, within their social, political and economic context. Gopee (2011) sees adult education in health care as collaborative in nature, the outcome aiming for the development of a responsible, autonomous practitioner.

Humanistic-based educational programmes are learner centred, encourage reflection on personal experience, give some freedom and choice as to content, call for collaborative learning and are delivered in a non-threatening, facilitative environment. These programmes are less likely to have detailed, pre-set objectives, and the goals may continually be in the process of modification. Maslow (1970) sees goal formation as a highly dynamic process occurring through the learner's unique interaction with their experience.

KEY POINTS

- Goals of learning need to be personally relevant to the learner.
- Personal learning is more important than knowledge acquisition.
- Self-awareness and self-evaluation are important to learning.
- Learning is a context-based natural process.

Comparing the three approaches

If we take a nursing handover from one shift to another as an example of clinical practice, we can illustrate how these different approaches to learning might be viewed (see Table 2.2).

Table 2.2 Learning to undertake 'handover' of a shift		
Behaviourism	**Cognitivism**	**Humanism**
The learner is 'conditioned' to undertake handover in a certain way that the rest of the profession has adopted in the locality (recognizes this, knows what to do, presents handover information as others do).	The learner is encouraged to develop a structure to their handover that can be adapted when they meet an unfamiliar situation (extrapolates and knows how to deal flexibly with the changed circumstance).	The learner comes across a situation where one of the patients whom they are discussing at handover appears distressed as their care is discussed.

These three learning theories tend to focus on the individual, and learning is seen as being dependent on experiences. (Further exploration of learning from experience is included in Chapter 6.)

Recently, there has been increased interest in learning as a social and situational process. Learning is enhanced through social participation. Observation and interaction within a social context, between people and the environment, is seen as the basis of learning, this is explored further later in the chapter.

TYPES OF KNOWLEDGE

The process of learning is affected by conceptions of knowledge. The following level descriptors (Baxter Magolda, 1992) have been offered as a way to pick out varying levels of learning.

1 **Absolutist** Knowledge is certain: 'I have to see what I'm learning about someone doing a patient assessment, and to know why I'm learning this'.

2 **Transition stage** Partial certainty and uncertainty: 'Being shown two methods of undertaking a patient assessment, which both appear successful, changes your views on the "right way" to handle a patient assessment'.

3 **Independent knowing** Learning is uncertain and everyone has their own beliefs: 'I take things in by watching others and hearing their opinions on how I might improve my patient assessment skills, but I decide what I want and what I don't want to do'.

4 **Contextual knowing** Knowledge is constructed and any judgement is made on the basis of evidence within a context: 'As I listen to the discussion regarding patient assessment, and think about my own experiences and others' viewpoints, I start to decide what I really think is important in this particular context'.

Reflective activity

Look at the level descriptors and the examples added, regarding patient assessment. Think about your own learning history. Can you identify a time in your life when your learning was absolutist, transitional, etc.? Did your age and the context that you were in at the time affect this?

Health care professionals require different kinds of knowledge. Evidence-based practice is a form of codified or empirical knowledge, defined by peer-reviewed research and published in books and journals, the 'gold standard' coming from randomized controlled trials. In order to approach care in an 'evidence-based' way, a practitioner needs to review the evidence available, thinking carefully and clearly about what makes most sense in influencing their clinical decisions. Wherever possible, scientific research that is relevant and properly conducted should be used. Evidence-based practice also means integrating individual clinical expertise with the best available external evidence.

Eraut (2000a) identifies cultural knowledge, located in space and time and interpreted differently by different groups, and personal knowledge which individuals bring to practical situations to help them think and perform. Phillips *et al.* (2000a) suggest that nurses make decisions through 'situated understanding' within practice settings.

There can be tensions between evidence-based practice and pragmatic practice. A knower's capacity to think and act is enhanced by the learning involved in making a 'scientific' concept available for use in a situation (Eraut, 2000b). However, even where research is reliable it may not be used in practice settings. The ability to make changes in practice is based on knowledge of the evidence available, and on learning from past experience. This is a complex art. The range of forms of knowledge and how they mix together is of great importance. It is recognized that Carper's (1978) empirical category of knowledge (she termed this 'scientific way of knowing') is supplemented by knowledge arising from:

- the art of performing clinical skills (aesthetic)
- the way nurses view and use themselves through being open to and focusing on the patient (personal)
- understanding the other person through recognizing one's own experiences (personal)
- handling practice dilemmas and making moral decisions through moment-to-moment judgements about what should be done, what is right, and what is responsible (ethical).

Observation of nurse–patient interactions reveals all of these in action. It is, therefore, unlikely that only one way of 'knowing' would be informing the way that a nurse acts.

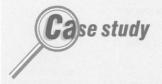

Case study

Forms of knowledge that inform professional working

Jane, a newly qualified staff nurse, is doing the post-operative observations for a woman who has returned after hernia surgery. A senior registered nurse is there watching her do the initial assess-ment. The newly qualified staff nurse is seeking approval for her work and for any omissions to be highlighted. She says, 'I'm not familiar with these forms.' The senior nurse shows her where to fill in the forms and sanctions her actions in disregarding certain parts of the form. She says, 'These are a bit more difficult. You could leave these as this is not applicable to day surgery – just make sure the wound is OK, and record the critical clinical data.'

What sorts of knowledge do you think are informing the junior and senior registered nurses' actions?

Aesthetics is the art of health care which involves seeing situations as a whole, not as component parts. It is the way that practitioners express and make their practice visible; through actions, bearing, conduct, attitudes, and interactions with patients. Carper (1978) suggests that aesthetics involves what is possible, not necessarily what is concrete, as the individual reflects on alternative courses of action. This way of knowing includes what is learnt as a result of professional experiences. It is how a practitioner selects from their total knowledge and builds upon a wealth of experience in order to perform the 'art-act' (Jacobs-Kramer and Chinn, 1988). Often, this process of engaging, interpretation, and envisioning is unconscious or intuitive and mainly portrayed in narratives of critical incidents and reflections on care decisions.

An appreciation of the importance of all these forms of knowledge partly explains the cynicism from some practitioners regarding the potential impact of evidence-based practice. However, in many situations common sense and opinions are not a good enough basis for making decisions or developing understanding. For example, in deciding which drug to prescribe the practitioner would need knowledge from all the domains identified by Carper (1978). Poor professional practice would be displayed if he or she prescribed a drug regimen that there was strong evidence to suggest was not appropriate. In addition, there is a need for informed consent about the drug treatment and to have an awareness of the individual and their ability to comply with the medical treatment regimen.

When you think about the ways in which context affects your learning, you may have identified the role of emotion in learning; recently, there has been increasing interest in the relationship between feelings and learning. Goleman (1995) coined the term 'emotional intelligence' to encompass the understanding and learning about self and others' emotions that guides effective decisions. Managing personal emotions in an intelligent way requires self-awareness, impulse control, persistence, motivation, empathy and social deftness. The ability to manage personal emotions and the emotions of others is seen as an important facet of health care practice. We explore how emotions can impact on care delivery further in Chapter 9.

LIFELONG LEARNING

Developing skills in order to continue to learn means that individuals become lifelong learners. Lifelong learning has been defined as a process of accomplishing personal, social and professional development (including formal, non-formal and informal learning) throughout the lifespan of the individual in order to enhance the quality of life of individuals and communities. Lifelong learning makes an assumption that learning takes place in all spheres of life, not just within educational institutes or in educational programmes. Lifelong learning is an important part of government policy related to a concern about the general skill and qualification levels of the economically active population. It is widely recognized that people will need continually to update and learn new skills if they are to remain competitive in the labour market. Titmus (1999) defines lifelong learning as the acquisition of learning skills for the immediate future, the ability to adapt such skills to meet the requirements of changing circumstance and applying learning to actions in a self-directed fashion.

Even though **self-directed learning** can be viewed as individual, self-directed adults use social networks and peer groups for emotional and educational support and guidance.

> **Self-directed learning**
> The process by which adults take control of their own learning; in particular, how they set their own learning goals, locate resources, decide on which learning methods to use and evaluate their progress

Over to you

Look at the characteristics of the lifelong learner outlined in the following table (adapted from ENB, 1994). In your own experience, and based on past learning, can you think of examples from your practice that might illustrate that you are already a lifelong learner?

Try to identify an example for each of the characteristics.

Innovative in your practice	
Flexible to changing demands	
Resourceful in your methods of working	
Able to work as a change agent	
Able to share good practice and knowledge	
Adaptable to changing health care needs	
Challenging and creative in your practice	
Self reliant in your way of working	
Responsible and accountable for your work	

- What characteristics did you find more difficult to write about?
- Why do you think that was?
- What does this tell you about your personal philosophy of practice?
- What could you do with the information you have just generated?

Gopee (2002) looked at human and social capital as facilitators to lifelong learning. He suggests that 'human capital' (the investment by employers and employees in personal and professional development activities) is interrelated with 'social capital' (the time, patience and teaching that colleagues invest in each other within the social group). Therefore, learning is not just the accumulation of individual 'human capital', but is a benefit to a community through the sharing of knowledge gained from continuous professional activities, conferences, workshops, by peers and expert practitioners (Gopee, 2002).

It has been argued that there is a significant and positive correlation between professional development and autonomy and recognition, role clarity, job satisfaction, quality of supervision, peer support and opportunities for learning (Hart and Rotem, 1995). Practitioners practise in an environment of constant change and, to help ensure that lifelong learning is occurring, they are required to develop and keep a portfolio of learning (termed 'a personal professional profile') and are encouraged to access clinical supervision.

CONTINUOUS PROFESSIONAL DEVELOPMENT

Being a lifelong learner is essential when developing professional practice. Before the 1990s, the majority of health care professionals' training focused on teaching routines and skills rather than on the ability to problem solve and rationalize the care given and exercise individual professional judgement. The increase in health care technology and the culture of constant change that is now synonymous with health care has influenced the need for increasingly competent and flexible professionals. Health care professionals have to provide some evidence of keeping themselves competent and up to date with their client care through continuous professional development (CPD).

CPD is:

> *... the way health professionals continue to learn and develop throughout their careers so they keep their skills and knowledge up to date and are able to work safely, legally and effectively.*
>
> *Health Professions Council 2011, p. 1*

CPD learning activities include:

- work-based learning, e.g. reflective practice, clinical audit, significant event analysis, user feedback, memberships of working groups/committees, journal club
- professional activity, e.g. member of a specialist interest group, mentoring, teaching, expert witness, presentations at conferences
- formal activity, e.g. courses, undertaking research, distance learning, planning and running a course
- self-directed learning, e.g. reading journals, articles, reviewing books, updating knowledge via the Internet, TV, press
- other activities, e.g. public service.

The way in which you take part in CPD will depend on your experiences and opportunities at work, profession or speciality, personal learning style, individual learning needs and the context of your practice.

Reflective activity

Take a blank sheet of paper and draw your professional time line starting when you first went into health care. Identify key learning events and changes to your professional working and experiences.

Nurses have been found to move frequently within the early years of their career, not in a 'migrant certificate gathering way', but getting good all round experience, actually creating pathways of professional development for themselves (Davies, 1995). Effective CPD has been linked with raised staff morale and increased motivation and is associated with staff retention (Mackereth, 1989). However, owing to methodological difficulties, there is a lack of conclusive evidence establishing a positive relationship between CPD and tangible improvements in patient care (Dowswell *et al.*, 1998; Wildman *et al.*, 1999), as many studies are based on the self-reports of learners (Smith and Topping, 2001). Community practitioners perceived that engaging in CPD would be beneficial to their motivation, and career succession (Banning and Stafford, 2008), however support from managers and peers was also considered crucial.

Smith and Topping's (2001) case study of a group of post-registration paediatric learners showed that nurses had taken the course for many reasons, including to improve their knowledge, improve their patient care, enhance career opportunities, improve their interprofessional relationships, increase their confidence and to help them act as a knowledge resource for others. Nurses' choice of course was underpinned by a need for the course to be relevant to their work and of personal interest. Although CPD was generally valued, individuals within this case study talked about their frustration in trying to put into practice changes in clinical care in a context where there were staffing shortages (Smith and Topping, 2001). A later study carried out by Hughes (2005) reported that the manager's leadership styles and their responsiveness to change were found to influence nurses' perceptions of CPD. It also affected their ability to reflect which had an impact on the application of learning to practice.

Continuous professional development is seen as essential for sustaining and improving the quality of professional work, and much CPD is based within practice (Eraut, 1994). Technological competence is often a key aim in undertaking post-registration courses, and nurses advocated acquiring this in the clinical context (Little, 1999). A specialist clinical course led to increased self-confidence in the nurses' standards of care and a more questioning attitude to the practice of others (Wood, 1998). Students' 'perceived benefit' from the course could, however, be no more than a 'feel good' factor on completion of a course (Wigens and Westwood, 2000). Specialist post-registration courses, assessed in practice, allow qualified practitioners to focus time on their own learning needs, giving unspoken 'permission' to ask questions of both nursing and medical colleagues (Little, 1999, p. 70).

Despite changes in course delivery and assessment, including problem-based learning and portfolio assessment of practice, some nurses have been found to have negative views of CPD. Courses available at post-registration level were viewed by some as lacking a comprehensive and responsive approach to practitioners' needs (DoH 1999; Robinson *et al.*, 2003). This was perhaps linked to a sense of CPD not being valued, in terms of the allocation of study time and financial support, and the perception that this affected career progression (Robinson *et al.*, 2003). It is argued that a flexible qualification system is required, with specialist qualifications that are updated when needed, and assessment systems that are capable of recording achievement beyond competence (Eraut, 1994).

SITUATED LEARNING

Reflective activity

Have you ever sat in a classroom listening to a lecture and thought to yourself, 'What relevance has this to the real world of practice?' Think about one of these times and try to identify why you were thinking this and whether, with the benefit of hindsight, your opinion has changed.

A possible reason why you were uninspired by that lecture is that the content was not easily remembered and seemed unrelated to your future working. Some theories of learning are based on what has been described as a 'content fetish' (Gee, 2004). From this stance, physiotherapy or nursing, for example, is composed of a set of facts and skills – a body of knowledge – and learning occurs when this information is taught to an individual and then tested. Conventional theories view learning as a process of individual internalization of knowledge; however, learning is also influenced by other people.

You have been introduced to the term situated learning and to situated understanding as a norm of everyday life. The question 'How are you today?' can mean different things in different contexts as people construct their own meaning from the social clues around them. The meaning of the communication and the expectations that it generates can be very different when 'How are you today?' is said in a ward setting, when someone appears distressed, compared with when it is used while passing an acquaintance in a hospital corridor. For some learning theorists (Lave and Wenger, 1991; Rogoff, 1990), any domain of knowledge is first and foremost a set of activities and experiences. For instance, nurses see, talk and do nursing when they are nursing and think about their interactions whilst nursing in a different way from non-nurses.

In developing the concept of the 'zone of proximal development' (ZPD), Vygotsky focused on the learning context as an important variable, shifting the emphasis from what has been learnt to learning capability (Cole *et al.*, 1978). Vygotsky suggested that a novice's development occurs through participation in activities beyond their competence with the assistance of skilled professionals who provide the 'scaffolding' for learning, and experts withdraw or 'fade' as increasing competency is shown by the novice (Rogoff, 1990).

There is a distinction between scientific knowledge and everyday concepts, and it is argued that maturity of learning is achieved when the scientific and everyday merge (Vygotsky, in Cole *et al.*, 1978). Engestrom (1994) expanded learning to include social transformation, covering all everyday actions from a wider historical and societal perspective. A key difference between Vygotsky's (in Cole *et al.*, 1978) and Lave and Wenger's (1991) views on social learning relates to the internalization of learning. Instead of viewing learning as internalization, Lave and Wenger take a more radical perspective, seeing learning as the result of increasing participation in communities of practice. (Refer back to Chapter 1 for a definition of communities of practice.) The development of situated learning was a response to trying to understand early forms of apprenticeship where students spent their time, often a number of years, gradually acquiring knowledge and skills from an expert.

> **Apprenticeship**
> A period of time working for a skilled person, often for low payment, in order to learn that person's skills

This form of learning was criticized as being context embedded, limited in scope, not sufficiently explicit, lacking in creativity, potentially out of date and as learning by rote. In a similar vein, clinical-based learning was traditionally a significant component of training for nursing and other health care professions but had been viewed as inferior to classroom-based higher education programmes. There is now increased acceptance of the situated nature of learning, and Lave and Wenger (1991) even go as far as to suggest that practical knowledge cannot be generalized or decontextualized.

Mikkelsen Kyrkjebø and Hage (2005) recognize that nursing students learn clinical practice from a range of communities of practice (we explore these further on p. 24) of very mixed quality. This can lead to the development of varying types of relationships between student health care practitioners and their clients; these relationships have been characterized as mechanistic, authoritative and facilitative (Suikkala and Leino-Kilpi, 2005).

- **Mechanistic relationship** Students focus on their own needs, intent on acquiring knowledge and technical skills. External factors such as the supervisor's daily routines and advice for performing physical tasks and aspects of care and treatment drive this type of relationship.
- **Authoritative relationship** Students assume what is best for the patient and problem-solve care; in some instances, patients are able to make decisions about their own care and treatment. Informal communications between the student and patient tend to be superficial.

- **Facilitative relationship** Patient's expectations and requirements for care and treatment govern student interactions. Students and patients know each other personally and the relationship could be described as close and warm (Suikkala and Leino-Kilpi, 2005).

The student's ability to develop a facilitative relationship with patients is affected by many factors, both individual and within the clinical milieu. The caring attributes of student nurses develop throughout their three years of training and through the varying cultures within their placements (Suikkala and Leino-Kilpi, 2005).

It has been suggested that various factors can promote or impede good student–patient relationships. These are identified within Table 2.3.

> **Clinical milieu**
> The physical and social aspects of the clinical environment: in fact, the totality of the surroundings

Table 2.3 Factors promoting or impeding good student–patient relationships	
Promoting factors	**Impeding factors**
Individual characteristics: • positive way of thinking, expectations and attitude • intellectual and interpersonal competence	Individual characteristics: • tendency to negativity or stereotyped expectations and attitudes • lack of intellectual and interpersonal competence
Patient-related factors: • positive frame of mind • favourable demographic and diagnostic characteristics	Patient-related factors: • tendency to negativity • unfavourable demographic and diagnostic characteristics
Length of time together: • patients' long hospital stays • students' long clinical placements • workload allocation is patient centred	Length of time together: • patients' short hospital stays • students' short clinical placements • workload high and task centred
Atmosphere: • role models of staff relationships with patients are good • supportive supervisory relationship • positive and encouraging feedback from clinical team	Atmosphere: • role models of staff relationships with patients are bad, lack of privacy during patient care and treatment • lack of supportive supervisory relationship • negative feedback from clinical team

(adapted from Suikkala and Leino-Kilpi, 2005, p. 350)

In the following account, a health professional identifies how she came to limit and define her nurse–patient relationship by learning through practice.

Health care professional

Registered nurse

During my training I was aware that I would occasionally get very attached to someone, particularly if I had done a lot of their care. I don't think you can opt out of becoming too involved, although during my training, we were told not to become too involved because we could become too stressed. I think that in the old-style training people were very worried that we'd get far too attached. I think I'm at a stage now where I became involved to a point. Since I qualified I have become more experienced at dealing with stress.

When you read what this nurse has to say about how she learnt about developing a nurse–patient relationship and about the comments from tutors and other health care staff to avoid 'getting too involved', what do you infer about the 'hidden curriculum' at that time? This type of 'general rule' appeared to be of little use to her when she first went into clinical placements.

Hidden curriculum
The unacknowledged, covert socializing processes of education that lead to the learning of cultural norms, values and beliefs

Marinker (1974) suggests that the hidden curriculum is learnt by observation and copying those around us. He stressed the importance of role models and the significance of mentors and supervisors reinforcing classroom messages through their clinical practice. The characteristics and behaviours of role models that were highly regarded by students include:

- effective practitioner
- learner- and patient-centred
- teamwork skills
- problem solver
- enthusiastic
- effective communicator
- leadership.

Allan *et al.* (2011) found that staff expect students to work while they learn. This could be at odds with the expectations of academic nurses, students had to negotiate their supernumery status.

KEY POINTS

- Situated learning contrasts with traditional classroom learning that involves knowledge presented in an abstract form or out of context
- Situated learning is a function of the activity, context and culture within which it occurs
- Learning can be incidental and requires social interaction and collaboration
- Knowledge needs to be presented in an authentic context

It is useful in understanding situated learning to look briefly at the concept of **professional socialization**.

Socialization theories focus on how the individual achieves membership of a group by internalizing its norms. Weidman *et al.* (2001) define professional socialization as the process by which people acquire the knowledge, skills, and disposition that makes them more effective members of a group, and higher education is a first step in this process. Through the process of acquiring prescribed knowledge, the student also learns about appropriate professional behaviour and attitudes. Individuals are developing professional values that guide their behaviours and define their sense of belonging to a professional group. The prescribed knowledge consists of the theoretical body of knowledge, methods and technology, and the interaction of all these elements produces professional language.

The socialization model presented by Weidman *et al.* (2001) has four components comprising professional socialization:

1 prospective students (background, predisposition)
2 professional communities (practitioners, associations)
3 personal communities (family, friends and employers)
4 novice professional practitioners.

According to this model, the ultimate outcome is the professional who has transformed their self-image, attitudes and thinking processes. Upon qualification, professionals embark on two more socialization processes: one into the organization that employs them and the second into their profession.

> **Professional socialization**
> Professional socialization is the process whereby newcomers to a profession acquire the values, attitudes, skills and knowledge that allow them to become a member of a professional subculture

Over to you

Read: Price, S.L (2008) Becoming a nurse: a meta-study of early professional socialization and career choice in nursing. *Journal of Advanced Nursing* 65(1): 11–19
Do you concur with the findings that early socialization is influenced by many factors?

Although professional socialization is an aspect of situated learning, Wenger (1998) suggests that education needs to be understood as changing identity in a lifelong process, not merely in terms of an initial period of socialization into a subculture, such as a profession. Learning through practice becomes a mutual development process between individuals and communities. There is a subtle difference between the imitation and internalization of norms and the construction of identities within communities of practice.

COMMUNITIES OF PRACTICE

At any given time, you belong to a range of communities of practice – at home, at work and in relation to your hobbies. These communities of practice are integral to your daily living: an example might be the members of a scout group where you act as the scout leader every Friday. The number and range of communities of practice vary throughout life, and what is learnt from these communities is personally transformative.

Reflective activity

Identify all the communities of practice that you belong to currently, and then compare this list to your own situation ten years ago. Think about how some of the communities of practice you were part of ten years ago have affected your learning.

Legitimate peripheral participation Legitimate peripheral participation is the process of increasing membership of a community of practice. It is legitimate because the learner is accepted as a potential community member working on the periphery of the community and acquiring knowledge through their practice with long-term community practice members. Learning occurs through the process of becoming a full participant

Situated learning is what individuals acquire by contributing to communities of practice, and communities continue to learn and refine their practice and to ensure continued membership. Lave and Wenger (1991) refer to an encompassing process called **legitimate peripheral participation** which is a defining characteristic of situated learning.

The term legitimate peripheral participation could, for example, relate to the experience of a student occupational therapist who is a 'newcomer'; in this context, the student's clinical supervisor could be viewed as an 'old-timer'. As time goes on, members of a community of practice start to understand the instances when 'old-timers' collaborate, collide and collude and also what is enjoyed, disliked, respected and admired in the group. Novices participate partially in examples of practice where these values are displayed. Over time, their depth of involvement grows and they redefine their identity. Novices learn actions, and a holistic explanation, from practitioners in the 'real world' setting and this helps them to handle some of the problems relating to the transference of learning.

It is suggested that nursing knowledge acquired in the authentic context has a better chance of being activated when needed in another situation (Lauder *et al.*, 1999). Looking at learning as being situated and encompassed within communities of practice does not mean that telling students to 'go out into practice' or just letting them loose into a clinical area is appropriate.

Reflective activity

Think about the first day that you went into your current or most recent practice setting. What things would you have liked to have known sooner, or been told about before you went into this clinical area?

You may have identified a number of things that you learnt through practice that with hindsight you would like to have been told by a mentor or colleague. However, it does not really work if you try to tell newcomers to a clinical area everything you think they will need, as many things cannot be put into words but are learnt through doing.

Health care settings can be stressful environments, and communities of practice can help staff to invent and maintain ways of coping. Wenger (1998) suggests that this can be accomplished through the resolution of conflict, reference to a communal memory, helping 'newcomers' to join, and determining 'what needs to be done'.

Communities of practice help in the management of difficult situations, such as high workload or interprofessional conflict. In the following excerpt, an operating department practitioner (ODP) talks about how things have changed within their professional learning and the impact on multidisciplinary working.

> **Communal memory**
> Communal memory involves the recollections and stories of past times and events that continue to be referred to by a community of people

Health care professional

Operating department practitioner

I think ODPs are changing for the better. It's nice to see us being given the opportunity to study for further degrees; if we want to it's there. It gives the theatre staff more credibility and allows us to stand our ground with doctors if we don't agree.

In the previous excerpt, an ODP indicates that there is often a level of conflict between the theatre-based staff and the surgeons. Although a community of practice sounds like it would be a site of harmony, it is understandable that within any group there will be multiple viewpoints.

Reflective activity

Think about the last three months and your working in a practice area over this time. How much of your learning was the consequence of time spent with a mentor/clinical supervisor? How much was the consequence of working with a range of staff within your clinical setting?

Communities of practice can serve as a 'living repository of knowledge', knowledge that can be 'sticky and leaky' and cross boundaries (Wenger *et al.*,

2002, p. 153). When you were reflecting on the past three months, some of your learning may well have been difficult to identify either in your thoughts or in writing, but you could perhaps have talked about it more easily with another person. The tacit aspects of knowledge are often the most valuable and can be shared through storytelling, conversation, coaching and learner support.

KEY POINTS

- Individuals and communities learn through their everyday practice
- Legitimate peripheral participation is the process whereby novices progress towards full membership of a community of practice
- Communities of practice are forums for situated knowledge, and can assist in resolving conflict

PROFESSIONAL KNOWLEDGE AND LEARNING

Knowledge based on community practice is professional knowledge. Understanding about professional knowledge has been limited by failure to conceptualize the different types of knowledge (Eraut, 1994). A professional is able to recognize 'situation and variation' (Benner, 1984), make competent judgements in unpredictable and complex situations, and apply knowledge and skills with the appropriate attitudes. Oakshott (1962) makes a distinction between 'technical knowledge' and 'practical knowledge'. Technical knowledge is written and codified, whereas practical knowledge is expressed only in practice and is learnt through experience in practice settings. Patel *et al.* (1999) suggest that there are two types of knowledge, factual knowledge that can be verbalized and intuitive knowledge that cannot. People acquire personal knowledge through experiences, either directly or vicariously. Personal knowledge is constructed through interaction with the wider context in which the experience occurs. In practice settings, all of these forms of knowledge are inextricably linked as a 'dynamic, integrated whole' (Williams, 1998, p. 28).

Over to you

Read: Hall, V. and Hart, A. (2004) The use of imagination in professional education to enable learning about disadvantaged clients. *Learning in Health and Social Care*, **3**(4), 190–202.

The sort of ideas expressed in the previous article question the traditional view of professional knowledge in which propositional knowledge gained from lectures and texts has to be reconstructed and applied in practice settings. Situated learning implies that knowledge and mastery of skills can only be acquired and successfully retained through practice in social, workplace contexts which are developing, changing and modifying. This rejects the separation of learning and the application of learning. If it is accepted that knowing is primarily about participating in a community of practice, then educational resources need to be directed at inventive ways of engaging students in meaningful practices, such as involving students in actions, discussions and reflections.

Practitioners should look critically at their own practice as part of their everyday routine, but they often seek to justify their practice rather than analyze it. The learner may well be able to view 'professional artistry' in action, but probably finds it more difficult to get to discuss what underpins this with a mentor or supervisor. Reflection can be a process for making explicit professionals' practical knowledge, and learners can process, interpret and generalize from their own experience and create mental frameworks to aid their understanding (Harrison *et al.*, 2002).

Situated learning is based on 'professional artistry', where only the principles or frameworks can be pre-determined and practitioners may for good 'context-specific' reasons choose to go beyond these principles (Fish and Coles, 1998). Schön (1983) discusses the importance of artistry within professional practice and questions the **technical rationality** model of professional knowledge as only applying to simplified problems and not the complex problems faced by professional practitioners.

The so called 'theory–practice gap' is seen as an artefact of the technical–rational view of professional education and can only exist where there is a belief that there is a clear separation of theoretical knowledge from practical knowledge (Fish and Coles, 1998, p. 45). Schön identified reflection-in-action, which occurs at the time of the encounter, and involves looking at our experience connecting with feelings and tacit knowledge, and reflection-on-action which occurs later after the encounter. Eraut (1994) is critical of Schön's (1983) notion of reflection-in-action, suggesting that it is really not reflection at all, but a single 'gut' judgement working in a reflexive rather than reflective fashion. Situated learning suggests that those who 'facilitate', 'coach' and 'mentor' have more relevance than those who purely 'teach' (Harrison *et al.*, 2002). There is also increased significance in informal learning gained through social relationships with colleagues, mentors, line managers and specialists (Eraut *et al.*, 1998).

Researchers who have focused on the importance of situated learning within nursing have mainly looked at this in relation to student nurses (Burkitt *et al.*, 2000; Cope *et al.*, 2000). Pre-registration student nurses talked about 'earning' social and professional acceptance which was not helped by short-duration placements (Cope *et al.*, 2000). Burkitt *et al.* (2000) identified two major problems facing student nurses: their location was within two communities of practice (higher education institute and clinical placements) and there were insufficiently strong links between the two. The multi-levelled

Technical rationality
Technical rationality views professional knowledge as being about empirical and scientific forms of evidence-based practice

nature of knowledge and practice needs to be reflected in the nursing curriculum through increased nurse lecturer involvement in practice and enhanced support for mentors (Burkitt *et al.*, 2000). At present, the multiple roles and multiple demands placed on experienced nurses leads to a process of successive interruptions and this, when combined with the fragmentation of practice placements and modularization, can reduce the meaningful learning opportunities for student nurses.

KEY POINTS

- There are many forms of knowledge used and developed within communities of practice, including knowledge constructed from personal experience, reflection and social interaction
- Situated learning requires practitioners to analyze critically their own and others' practice as part of their everyday working
- Situated clinical learning is best supported through facilitation, coaching and mentorship, rather than through 'traditional' clinical teaching
- The importance of dynamic and problem/solution-focused professional artistry should be acknowledged in health care practice

COMMUNITY OF PRACTICE DEVELOPMENT

There is no doubt that the clinical milieu is full of rich learning experiences, and that learning is more meaningful if the student participates actively within a clinical team whilst on placement. Six factors have been identified as playing key roles: staff (registered and assistants)–student relationships, the manager, commitment to teaching, patient relationships, student satisfaction and hierarchy/ritual (Dunn and Hansford, 1997). Pearcey and Elliott (2004) found that the culture of the clinical area impacted both on the student learning experience and also on their impressions of their chosen profession. It is more than just the availability of time that imparts a caring, better culture: the whole philosophy of the clinical team affected the atmosphere (Pearcey and Elliott, 2004).

Student

Third-year student

It is really refreshing to be on a placement where there is good morale and they're well staffed. When the team aren't particularly negative and are happy about their care delivery, it can make a difference to whether you want to stay on the course and qualify. My experience on this placement has made me change my mind about carrying on to work in this field when I qualify.

Community-building skills are displayed through practitioners' warmth and concern for others and the ambience of an active community. One of the most important features of any workplace or community context is the people with whom one interacts – colleagues, friends, customers, clients and acquaintances. An important way, therefore, of improving clinical learning is through investing time and energy into developing team relationships, sharing common objectives and needs to be fulfilled. A range of factors has been found to help in the development of clinical teams and the increasing movement towards group needs. These include:

- personal commitment
- sharing a common goal
- clarity of roles
- good lines of communication
- institutional support
- leadership (Wigens, 2005).

The clinical/ward manager plays a vital role; Smith's (1992) research described the ward sister/charge nurse as the 'architect' of nursing work who sets the emotional and organizational agenda of the ward. A clinical leader in one case study identified how important her own and other staff's CPD had been in influencing improvements in her clinical area (Wigens, 2004). Clinical leadership is linked to a commitment to CPD and lifelong learning, and senior staff acted as role models for this.

The leader also has an impact on the pre-registration learner's experience. The opportunities offered by different placement areas can be very diverse given the fact that on the face of it little differs from a service perspective. One thing that does however differ is the workforce and the team in it. Two essential components of effective teams are that they have an effective leader and clear communication between all. Northouse (p. 3, 2009) says that leadership 'is a process whereby an individual influences a group of individuals to achieve a common goal'. He says that influence is the very essence of leadership and if absent, leadership doesn't exist. So the underlying mental model and priorities of the leader will inevitably impact on the team. Students have reported that the leadership style and particularly the ward sister's attitude to supernumery status can have an effect on its implementation (McGowan, 2006, p. 1101), 'where sister led the staff were sure to follow'.

Health care professional

Staff nurse – day surgery unit

In our unit here we're given a lot of opportunity to do things because we've got a really good sister who makes sure that we are keeping ourselves up to date. You feel that you want to, because she studies too.

In health care, emphasis has been placed on developing 'transformational leadership', which involves paying attention to the needs of individuals and the group processes, ensuring feedback on performance, developing a stable and trusting workforce, supporting networking and technology and using emotional intelligence (McCormack *et al.*, 2002). Transformational leadership transposes individual beliefs and values into collective beliefs and values so that they become taken for granted. Stordeur *et al.* (2001) suggest that nurses who experience an imbalance between efforts expended at work and the reward obtained are more likely to be emotionally exhausted, and that leadership roles can buffer the effects of a demanding work environment by maintaining a supportive leadership style. Transformational leaders motivate staff to do more than initially expected and are change agents that transmit a sense of mission, instil faith and respect and treat each employee as an individual (Stordeur *et al.*, 2001).

Situational leadership is based on the assumption that there is no one singularly successful leadership style, and that a variety of effective leadership styles should be used, dependent on the context. Some of the skills identified for being an effective facilitator or leader include being a source of clinical advice, having local credibility and understanding of the 'system', and being pragmatic and motivated (Harvey *et al.*, 2002).

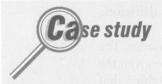

Case study

Clinical leadership and its impact on learning

Sian, a community midwife, identified that many teenage women in her clinical locality were not attending antenatal classes regularly, and so did not receive proper care or midwifery support. When Sian discussed this with the community midwifery team, they agreed that this was a priority area to be tackled and also that, as well as accessing these expectant mothers more actively and offering antenatal support in a different way to capture this group, they should work with other stakeholders. Sian set up a group to work on improving antenatal care for teenage mothers, involving user representation, staff from mainstream education, local colleges, adult education centre, Brook advisory centre, health visitors, school nurses and youth services. The group decided that they wanted to work on a way to help teenagers who were pregnant make healthy informed choices about their life-style, and therefore their babies' health (e.g. low birthweight is indicative of a tendency to coronary disease in later life, DoH, 2000a). The stakeholders and the midwifery clinical team developed a local resource pack for teenage mothers and a guidance tool for education and health care professionals to use with this antenatal group.

When the midwifery clinical team talked about Sian they described her in the following ways:

● She's inspirational and motivational – she just 'goes for it'.

● She holds on to her vision, even when times get tough, and you can always count on her to do 'the right thing'.

● She is able to listen to other people's views, and to work across boundaries to build relationships.

Having looked at this particular case, can you identify any other things you might add to describe this successful leader?

Have you come across a clinical leader like this within your practice, and did their leadership skills have an impact on the clinical learning environment?

Although the midwife in the previous case study did refer to research findings, her decision-making was not just based on this. The knowledge developed by individual health care practitioners through their decision-making and experience is different from contemporary published scientific knowledge. Networking can involve sharing of knowledge through person-to-person contact, and oral story telling, which is particularly well developed in health care, can be a way of communicating knowledge, as practitioners find it easier to talk about good practice, rather than write about it (Burke and Smith, 2000).

Practitioners do not apply research findings in a simple deductive process: they need time to think, translate and particularize research findings (Titchen, 2000). Further examination of practice development is included in Chapter 6.

Strategies for making non-research knowledge explicit include reflection, discussion of critical incidents in the clinical setting, enhancement of evaluative cultures, peer review, and clinical supervision (LeMay, 1999). Making time for staff discussions about the effectiveness of clinical practice and clinical supervision/mentorship within the setting could address concerns and lead to continual improvement.

Learning organizations should pay attention to the needs of individuals and groups as well as to the organizational systems. Wenger and colleagues' (2002) exploration of communities of practice relationships to their employing organization identified five main relationships:

1 unrecognized or invisible
2 bootlegged, and only visible informally to the circle of people in the know
3 legitimized and officially sanctioned as valuable
4 strategic and widely recognized as central to organizational success
5 transformative, and capable of redefining its environment.

As clinical teams develop, they may progress through these levels of relationships within their institutions. What level would you choose to describe the ward team who attended the staff meeting in the following clinical caseload?

CLINICAL CASE LOAD

At a ward staff meeting, the following suggestions were made for improving the quality of clinical learning experiences for qualified practitioners and students (adapted from Palmer *et al.*, 2005, Table 2).

1 Students need to undertake complete care interventions for their patients, as much as is feasible given their skills level.
2 All staff should be provided with information on the current skill level of students and their learning objectives for the clinical area.

3 Students should work the same shift pattern and attend all clinical team discussions, so that they are integrated members of the health care delivery team.

4 All mentors/supervisors should be provided with information on how to effectively mentor students and new staff to the area.

Do you agree with the suggestions? Would you add any further suggestions to be discussed in the staff meeting?

A hidden curriculum of observed behaviour and interactions and the overall norms and culture of a student's training environments shape the values, attitudes and professional identity of future health care professionals. Professional identity is integrated with a personal sense of identity and involves the individual's having a feeling of being able to practise with skill, being able to articulate clearly their commitment to their profession, and taking responsibility for their own actions, whilst maintaining an awareness of their attributes and limitations (Ohlen and Segesten, 1998).

As individuals are members of many communities of practice, identity can be multi-dimensional and arises in interaction with others (Sarup, 1996). Situated learning is personally meaningful. Motivation, activity and learning are related to positive self-esteem and identity, and the individual health care practitioner is shaped by their relationship to their community of practice. For example, membership of a nursing community is inextricably linked with individual motivations to nurse and engagement through development of a 'professional identity'. This 'professional identity' motivates learning and working and is not always 'switched off' when a nurse leaves work (Wigens, 2004). Although there is a sense of being a member of a 'common nursing profession', over time the nurse also becomes aligned to the health care context. There is internalization of the values, knowledge, skills, norms and culture occurring in relation to nursing, but also towards the speciality in which the nurse works.

Being able to outline the differences between the chosen speciality and the professional role to others is part of nurses' striving for positive social identity. Membership of groups, cliques and sub-groups within the nursing workplace is valuable both for mutual support and help, and it also increases power, allowing nurses to gain control and resist unwanted change. Nurses consider reflective discussions with colleagues during group supervision as important in the development of their professional identity and for community building (Ohlen and Segesten, 1998).

KEY POINTS

- Clinical learning is most effective within a clinical milieu where practitioners are engaged, warm, reflective and work together with active concern for staff and patients
- It is worth investing time and energy in the development of a community of practice, including its knowledge base
- Transforming situational leadership is vital in ensuring effective clinical learning opportunities
- Communities of practice influence the professional identities of both qualified practitioners and students

POSSIBLE PROBLEMS WITHIN COMMUNITIES OF PRACTICE

Further examination of how communities of practice can be fostered appears in the online bonus feature for this chapter. However, within any community of practice there is a risk that innovators will be 'held hostage' to the experience of the 'elders', with statements such as, 'We've tried that before and it didn't work' (Wenger, 1998, p. 85). Because of this, a community of practice can become so insular that its members become unable to register other viewpoints, and this can become an obstacle to learning and change (Wenger, 1998, p. 98). Members of a community of practice, like any social group, can specialize, gain reputation, distinguish, create different statuses, join cliques and share gossip. Enthusiasm can lead to arrogance, and a community can become dependent on one leader. Alternatively, a community can become marginalized and not be taken seriously (Wenger *et al.*, 2002).

In leaving professional learning totally to 'legitimate peripheral participation' there is a possibility that practice could become outmoded, inherited from 'old-timers' with a lack of new ideas to stimulate changes in practice. Lave and Wenger (1991) argue that stagnation will not occur, however, because the focus of learning continues through the 'community of practice' and knowledge is continuously created.

Reflective activity

Have you ever been in a clinical setting and felt that practice had become outmoded and was stagnating? What factors did you feel had the most impact on this situation?

An under-developed aspect of Lave and Wenger's (1991) theory of situated learning is the role given to reflection on practice (Maudsley and

Strivens, 2000), and it would be a good idea to link your understanding of communities of practice to the discussion on reflection incorporated in Chapter 6. Although Lave and Wenger (1991, p. 109) identify 'talking about' practice and relating stories as a form of memory and reflection, they say little about the way that stories are regularly revised to take account of changing needs, aspirations and motivations.

Some critics claim that Lave and Wenger's theory is too all-encompassing, with its assertion that all learning takes place within the social setting, and argue for a distinction between social learning and individual learning, with individual learning taking place independently of the social context. It is alleged that one risk in over-advocating the value of situated learning is that it undermines the role of professional education that is delivered within educational institutes with the expectation that this will be transferred to practice. Perhaps the problem is that some interpretations of Lave and Wenger's work have incorrectly concluded that they are claiming that knowledge learnt in a classroom setting cannot be used in practice. My view is that the social and individual are so intertwined that you cannot just focus on the individual. The individual aspects of clinical learning are explored within the next chapter.

KEY POINTS

- There is a risk with communities of practice that they can become insular, marginalized and less open to change
- The concept of communities of practice needs to be further developed with regard to the role of reflection and frameworks for participation

RAPID RECAP

Check your progress so far by working through each of the following questions.

1 What are the key differences between outcome-based and process-based learning?

2 List the key principles underpinning:

   (a) behaviourist theories of learning

   (b) cognitive theories of learning

   (c) humanistic theories of learning.

3 Explain the concepts 'lifelong learning' and 'continuous professional development'.

4 Why is it useful to be able to document learning through practice?

5 Define the term 'hidden curriculum' within health care professional education

6 Explain in your own words what 'legitimate peripheral participation' means

7 Identify five factors that help the development of a community of practice clinical team.

If you have difficulty with any of these questions, read through the section again to refresh your understanding before moving on

CHAPTER 3

MENTORSHIP IN NURSING AND MIDWIFERY

LEARNING OBJECTIVES

By the end of this chapter you should be able to:

● identify the roles that support learners within practice

● recognize the expectations of your professional body

● appreciate the common challenges encountered by all health care professionals when supporting learning in practice

● develop an awareness of the strategies to support an underachieving learner

Bonus features for this chapter available on the book's website

INTRODUCTION

The relationship between the student health care practitioner and the practitioner responsible for their practice-based learning is often one of novice to expert and can be called different things depending on the professional group. For instance, nurses call this a mentorship relationship, whereas occupational therapists would term it clinical supervision. The transition from novice learner through to advanced beginner (Benner, 1984) and onwards sees the learner becoming more actively involved in setting the agenda. Although, within this chapter, we have looked at supporting practice-based learning for students under the heading 'mentorship', the content applies across professions and encompasses practice teacher working.

Although mentorship and models of professional support are given separate chapters within this book, the content relating to particular skills is relevant to all these facilitation roles. Giving and receiving feedback (included within the mentorship section), role-modelling (included within the preceptorship section), and challenging another's practice (which is incorporated in the clinical supervision section), are equally applicable to mentorship, preceptorship and clinical supervision.

A SHORT HISTORY

Nursing mentorship was changed in line with the Department of Health's 'Making a Difference' strategy for nursing in 1999 (Walsh 2010), subsequently nursing and midwifery pre-registration programmes were required to become 50 per cent theory and 50 per cent practice. This coincided with the United Kingdom Central Council for Nursing, Midwifery and Health Visiting's review of Nurse Education 'Fitness for Practice' (UKCC, 1999) which stressed the need to emphasize the role of the mentor (Walsh, 2010).

Mentors are influential in shaping a learner's practice and therefore influence 'practice wisdom' for many years (Price, 2004). The classic concept of a mentor, used in other contexts, refers to a trusted counsellor who maintains this relationship over a period of time, and mentor relationships were originally viewed as growing between two individuals over two to 15 years. In contrast, a mentor who oversees practice learning in one placement for a student practitioner does so usually for no more than 10–12 weeks. Nevertheless, the term 'mentor' is used within nursing and midwifery for the placement clinical supervisor, whereas other health care professions more commonly use the term 'clinical supervisor'.

The impact that an effective mentoring experience can have on the learner should not be underestimated. In producing the 'Standards to Support Learning and Assessment in Practice' (2006) the Nursing and Midwifery Council (NMC) sought to strengthen the practice of mentorship. The role of the mentor is regarded as pivotal in pre-registration preparation (Moseley and Davies, 2007), and increasingly recognized over the last ten years (Bray and Nettleton, 2007). Most registered nurses and midwives perform this role at some point in their career.

Education in nursing and midwifery can be considered from three simple perspectives;

- that those nurses and midwives practising should be doing so in an effective and efficient manner
- that those at the point of registration should be competent to be there
- that programmes preparing them should be appropriate to the context of care.

These perspectives encompass regulation, quality assurance, an appreciation of the service and an awareness of the needs of the service user.

ROLES AND RESPONSIBILITIES

Public expectations of health care professionals are high; therefore it is not an unreasonable expectation that the programmes that prepare registered practitioners perform this task in a suitable manner. In these programmes 50 per cent of the assessment is done by practitioners in the clinical environment. Duffy (2004) found that some students pass practice assessments when there is in fact some doubt about their clinical competence and they may then subsequently go on to achieve registration.

Efficacy
producing the desired result, in the case of a mentor being an effective mentor and carrying out the role as required.

In essence then the efficacy of mentorship is vital if future practitioners are to be fit for purpose and practice. The quality of the student–mentor relationship has a direct influence on the development of the novice practitioner, and this is likely ultimately to influence patient care. Wilkes (2006) considers the relationship crucial in light of the assessing role particularly. In a review of the literature she found that students view a 'good mentor' as being someone who has a positive attitude and is patient and friendly, reflecting an emotional need for the relationship to be nurturing.

Key components of the mentor role

Some practitioners seem inherently to possess the skills and qualities for mentorship, whereas others need to work on some areas: for example, a key skill is the ability to negotiate learning, and a mentor may need to work on the ability to challenge the learner's goals for their practice.

Reflective activity

- What does the term 'mentor' mean to you?
- What qualities and skills do you think an effective mentor should have?
- How does a mentor benefit from taking on this role?
- As a student, what would you like your mentor to do?

The key components of the role of the mentor are identified here. Are these in line with what you thought during the last reflective activity?

Role of the mentor

- Identifying the needs of the learner
- Advising learners on the type of support available
- Providing guidance about facilities and learning resources in the organization
- Following up comments from other staff about students who are performing poorly or whose conduct is unacceptable
- Referring students with particular problems to the appropriate agencies
- Carrying out assessment of learning
- Completing the practice of assessment recording on completion of the placement

Mentorship of students is often viewed as an integral part of the qualified health care practitioner's role. Some professions require additional education before the practitioner can formally take on this role: for example, Preparation for Mentorship programmes of study. Others, however, may deem that sufficient knowledge of the role can be imparted over a study day. In either case, mentors should develop a good understanding of the principles covered within the module through which the learner is progressing during their clinical placement. They need to be knowledgeable about the learning outcomes, desired competencies and the forms of evidence which can be used to show achievement of these.

The NMC describes a mentor as someone who has successfully completed an approved mentor preparation programme and achieved the required knowledge, skills and competence necessary to undertake the role (NMC, 2008) stating that:

> *Mentors are responsible and accountable for:*
>
> - *Organizing and co-ordinating student learning activities in practice.*
> - *Supervising students in learning situations and providing them with constructive feedback on their achievements.*
> - *Setting and monitoring achievement of realistic learning objectives.*
> - *Assessing total performance – including skills, attitudes and behaviours.*
> - *Providing evidence as required by programme providers of student achievement or lack of achievement.*
> - *Liaising with others (e.g. mentors, sign-off mentors, practice facilitators, practice teachers, personal tutors, programme leaders) to provide feedback, identify any concerns about the student's performance and agree action as appropriate.*
> - *Providing evidence for, or acting as, sign-off mentors with regard to making decisions about achievement of proficiency at the end of a programme.*
>
> *NMC, 2008 p. 19*

According to Casey and Clark (2011) the NMC's professional definition of a mentor is different from a generic definition, there is a responsibility for assessment and therefore judging the quality of the student's practice. The partnership must remain professional with clear boundaries that ensure the balance between support and assessment.

A clinical team that views student learning as a priority may choose to identify one staff member who takes the lead in working with the educational institute and its staff. This role has sometimes been called an 'educational link'; the chosen person is also likely to be a 'sign-off' mentor (someone who determines assessment to practice at the end of the pre-registration programme) or a practice teacher. This link role should improve communication between the higher education institute and the clinical team, and will help co-ordination and information sharing.

One way of assessing the potential of an individual to be a mentor/clinical supervisor/practice teacher would be to self-assess their skills and qualities using the range of 'ideal' types identified through research (Darling, 1984). The 'functions' model of mentorship, developed by Darling (1984), found 14 main dimensions:

- a **model** the student can value and admire and may wish to emulate
- a **visioner** who is enthusiastic about opportunities or possibilities and inspires interest
- an **energizer** who makes the profession fascinating and is enthusiastic and dynamic
- an **investor** who spends a lot of time with the learner, spots potential and capabilities and can hand over responsibility
- a **supporter** who is willing to listen, is warm and caring and is available in times of need
- a **standard-pusher** who is very clear about what level of performance is required and prompts the learner to achieve it
- a **teacher-coach** who can instruct about setting priorities, help to develop interpersonal skills, give guidance on patient problems and encourage learning from experience
- a **feedback giver** who can offer both positive and negative feedback and help the student to examine the things that go wrong
- an **eye opener** who inspires interest in research and is able to facilitate understanding of wider issues, such as Trust politics and departmental issues
- a **door opener** who includes the student in discussions and offers the student opportunities to be involved in new areas of practice
- an **idea bouncer** who not only discusses issues, problems and goals, but also allows the learner to present and argue ideas
- a **problem solver** who helps the student to figure out and try out new ideas and can analyze strengths and create ways to use them for the benefit of the profession or the job
- a **career counsellor** who gives guidance and support in career planning
- a **challenger** who questions opinions and beliefs and forces the student to examine decisions (adapted from Darling, 1984).

It is useful to consider the fact that the importance and emphasis of each role depends on the individual students, and at which stage of development and learning they are; it is the skill of the mentor to recognize and react appropriately in order to optimize the student's experience and progress (Ali and Panther, 2008).

Over to you

Assess yourself in terms of these characteristics:

Table 3.1 Characteristics of a mentor (adapted from Darling, 1984)				
Characteristic	**This is a particular strength of mine**	**I can offer this**	**This is not a particular strength**	**I don't want this role**
Model				
Visioner				
Energizer				
Investor				
Supporter				
Standard-pusher				
Teacher-coach				
Feedback giver				
Eye opener				
Door opener				
Idea bouncer				
Problem solver				
Career counsellor				
Challenger				

Review the boxes you have ticked and think about what areas you need to work on to improve your future mentorship/supervisory work.

The 'functions' approach can be helpful when thinking about mentorship, but it is perhaps easier to consider the key qualities and skills of a 'good' mentor.

Reflective activity

Recall a mentor or senior practitioner whom you identified in the past as a role model for your working in practice. What made this person a positive or inspiring influence?

When we asked a group of student nurses on placement in one NHS Trust, these were the factors that they suggested were displayed by 'good' mentors'.

Qualities of a 'good' mentor/clinical supervisor

- Prepared to allocate time and energy to this role
- Well-trained and supported themselves
- Has a good sense of humour and is patient, not expecting all students at the same stage in training to be the same in their clinical achievements
- Up to date with recent initiatives and prepared to be flexible and innovative
- Competent in the core skills of coaching, counselling, facilitating, giving feedback and networking
- Interested and willing to help others
- Willing to learn and can see the potential benefits of taking on the role
- Can record progress and identify the level of learning
- Able to help learners who have problems/difficulties
- Able to act as a role model

The mentor that you thought about in the last reflective activity may well have been an excellent clinical practitioner, but there is a risk that a role model may be chosen by novice practitioners without questioning their standards of practice (Andrews and Roberts, 2003). Clinical expertise is not necessarily synonymous with mentorship expertise, as the qualities and skills required are subtly different. In addition, workload pressures within senior clinical roles may adversely affect the delivery of the mentorship role. Finding dedicated time to offer learners can be a great challenge: often, mentorship is relegated to taking place 'after the work has been done'. It is crucial that the individual desires to take on the mentorship role. Doing so because there is the expectation that they should, owing to its inclusion in a job description, or in order to gain promotion is a poor basis for enthusiastic and committed learner support (Andrews and Chilton, 2000).

The necessity of practice learning is irrefutable. The management of the balance between needs of the service and education of the future workforce needs to be responsive and dynamic. The clinical environment contains many opportunities for the learner, and is enhanced by active participation, however effective mentorship is only measured by student achievement (Andrews and Roberts, 2003).

Influencing factors in the mentoring role

Occasionally an *ad hoc* mentoring approach can occur as a result of staff shortages and annual leave (McGowan, 2006), and when this happened learning needs were perceived as being compromised as service demands increased. However Myall *et al.* (2008) found that students recognize that there were <u>organizational and contextual constraints</u> placed on mentors' efficacy which affected the quality of placement experience. This places all stakeholders in a dilemma over the consequences of their decision making and prioritizing.

McGowan (2006) discovered, during his study on the perceptions of undergraduate pre-registration students regarding supernumery status, that students felt that there was a correlation between the positive approach to learning and the experience of the learner and the leadership/management style. This appears to show that there is a variance in the efficacy of mentorship which is dependent on the leader. Spouse (1998) identified learning to nurse as a complex interaction of affective, practical and cognitive factors adding that the nature and quality of the clinical environment influences the integration of them all. The clinical environment constantly changes in line with issues such as staffing, workload, practice delivery and development, and this complexity is combined with the fact that although mentors might be willing to take on their role, often they are not supported by resources to undertake this endeavour (Edmond, 2001).

Whilst the mentor retains accountability and responsibility for their student they are only part of the context: the clinical leader; clinical context and learning environment; the Higher Education Institution; and service provided by the placement, all contribute to the experience. However, the interaction between the mentor and student remains central and of great significance.

Nurses are more likely to take on a clinical facilitation role if they have undertaken further studies themselves, balancing a sense of responsibility for 'good' nursing care with developing the learning culture. Mentors share their responsibility for learning with other qualified staff, making the 'space' for learning, and asking for confirmation of their student's learning progression (Ohrling and Hallberg, 2001a).

Relationships

We are building up a picture that the quality of the mentor-student relationship influences the progression of the student, and as students learn from their mentors they move towards practising independently under indirect supervision (Spouse, 2003). Spouse suggests that 'good' mentorship comprises four characteristics:

- befriending
- planning
- confederacy (acting as an ally)
- coaching.

A caring and trusting relationship between a mentor and student produces the most effective learning in clinical practice, and a student who is not actively 'befriended' can feel isolated and lacking in direction (Spouse, 2003). The characteristics Spouse identifies are displayed through:

- planning prior to the expected start date of the mentee
- welcoming the mentee in a warm manner and developing rapport
- planning their time and rosters to ensure consistency of mentorship
- explaining their actions and the rationale underpinning these
- directly supporting the student when they undertake a care practice for the first time.

Mentors vary in their approach to their mentorship role, with the outcome that students receive mixed experiences ranging from highly motivated through to disinterested (Pearcey and Elliot, 2004). Failure to live up to students' expectations of a mentor can be the greatest cause of disappointment in clinical practice learning for students (Pearcey and Elliot, 2004). Mentors may meet learners who appreciate the need for mentorship in a general sense, but who are not really sure of their real value. This can be helped not only by negotiating and facilitating learning but also by agreeing the 'ground rules' of the mentor–mentee relationship.

There can be negative consequences from mentoring, and it has been suggested that there is a fine line between mentor and tormentor (Feldman, 1999). There are potential pitfalls if either party enters the relationship with unrealistic expectations of time commitment or objective benefits. There can be toxic mentors, toxic protégés and toxic environments (Feldman, 1999), and any one of these three elements can adversely affect the balance within the mentoring relationship. A mentor–mentee relationship may be dysfunctional if the needs of either party are frustrated by the relationship, if the cost of the relationship outweighs its benefit, or if specific behaviours of one sabotage the working of the other.

EVIDENCE BASE

Read: Levett-Jones *et al.* (2009) Staff-student relationships and their impact on nursing students' belongingness and learning. *Journal of Advanced Nursing*, **65**(2): 316–324.
   Think about your experiences, how do they influence your future engagement with learners?

Levett-Jones *et al.* (2009) found that a positive approach can be seen as important if students are to feel accepted, included and valued. In the study they identified that students said that if they felt part of the culture and team, then all nurses regardless of whether they were responsible for mentoring also supported their learning. Building this relationship can be as simple as greeting your student with a smile and making that connection on a basic respectful human level.

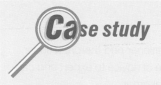

Mentorship

Shakeel was struggling to encourage his mentee Sandra to become interested in learning more about the drugs used within the cardiac care ward. However, Sandra seemed to feel that Shakeel was testing her knowledge base, and said, 'We haven't learnt about this at college yet'. Shakeel decided to start simply, by using examples from everyday practice on the ward. He was arranging the discharge of a patient that day, and the patient was going home on the latest ACE inhibitor*. Shakeel explained that he would need to discuss how the drug works, the possible problems and side effects with the patient. He asked Sandra to think about what she could do to prepare herself to help with

this information giving prior to discharge. Sandra was encouraged to look up drugs from this group, e.g. Captopril, in the British National Formulary. Shakeel and Sandra discussed what other options there would be for finding out the information required, such as pharmacist, doctor, and other sources of drug information. Using this 'real' situation reinforced the understanding that, to work effectively in practice, a medication knowledge base is required and allowed the mentee to appreciate the need for lifelong learning regarding medication management.

What other approaches could a mentor take to a mentee who appears uninterested in furthering their learning on an aspect of practice?

*An ACE inhibitor is an angiotensin-converting enzyme inhibitor that reduces peripheral vascular resistance via blockage of the angiotensin-converting enzyme. This action reduces the myocardial oxygen consumption, thereby improving cardiac output and moderating left ventricular and vascular hypertrophy.

The NMC (2008) advises that mentors spend a minimum of 40 per cent of student's placement learning time (nominally 15 working hours in a full week) with their mentee undertaking either direct or indirect supervision. Myall *et al.* (2008) found that students felt that the amount of time that they spent with their mentors affected the quality of the learning environment. Particularly important was whether they were able to work with their mentor during the first week of the placement, and for two or three shifts in each subsequent week. Duffy (2004) suggests that the amount of time spent with a mentee may contribute to a reduction in mentor's ability to fail students. Glasper (2010) considers this time factor is vital, as accurate judgements need to be made. When the staff roster or work plan is being devised, mentor/clinical supervisor allocation should be taken into account (Price, 2004). Students should be identified on the roster with their shifts clearly linked to that of their mentor. Arrangements should be made for supervision in the absence of the mentor. Even when this proves difficult, some mentors are able to support learners within the limited time available because they plan learning activities, work alongside the learners when possible, and delegate mentee support through giving their colleagues associate mentor roles. It is, therefore, important to look to the wider clinical team within the mentor's health care setting as partners in supporting student learning.

KEY POINTS

- The relationship between the student health care practitioner and the practitioner responsible for their practice-based learning is often one of novice to expert and can be called different things depending on the professional group
- This process of 'mentorship' is an influential aspect of practice learning
- The role of the mentor encompasses a variety of dimensions which all contribute to the learning experience
- Challenges to the implementation of the role need to be recognized and addressed
- Developing a positive relationship is an essential element

ADHERING TO NMC REGULATORY STANDARDS

This NMC 'Standard to Support Learning and Assessment in Practice (2006) sets the standards and outcomes for mentors, practice teachers and teachers of nurses, midwives and specialist community public health nurses. It was originally published in October 2006 for implementation from September 2007 as the 'Standards to Support Learning and Assessment in Practice'. A second edition, containing clarification and interim circulars, was published in May 2008. This latter edition will be used as the current reference point.

The standards demonstrate the significance placed on the practice component of programmes and provides guidance for registered practitioners and organizations (Andrews *et al.*, 2010). There is a single developmental framework to support learning and assessment in practice which defines and describes the knowledge and skills registrants need to apply in practice when they support and assess students undertaking NMC approved programmes that lead to registration or a recordable qualification on the register. This contains the outcomes related to each of the four stages identified here which are mapped to the eight mentor domains (see Table 3.2).

Table 3.2 Stages in NMC standards			
Stage 1	Stage 2	Stage 3	Stage 4
NMC registrant	Mentor	Practice Teacher	Teacher

The standards are underpinned by five principles which underpin the identification of those nurses and midwives who are suitable to make judgments about whether a student has achieved the required standards of proficiency for safe and effective practice. Mentors MUST:

A   be on the same part or sub-part of the register as that which the student is intending to enter.

B have developed their own knowledge, skills and competency beyond that of registration through Continuous Professional Development (either formal or experiential learning, as appropriate to their support role).

C hold professional qualifications equal to or at a higher level than, the students they are supporting and assessing.

D have been prepared for their role to support and assess learning and have met NMC defined outcomes – where possible achieving these outcomes in practice, supporting interprofessional learning and where relevant in academic settings.

E Nurses and midwives who have completed an NMC approved teacher preparation programme may record their qualification on the NMC register.

The mentorship preparation programme is delivered at a minimum academic level 2, through a minimum of ten days' learning inclusive of five days protected time, and is normally completed within three months (NMC, 2008). The mentor is required to have studied at the same or higher level than the student to ensure that the mentor's knowledge and skills are at a level where the complexity of practice assessment for the individual student is handled effectively (NMC, 2008). A mentor should be able to demonstrate an understanding of the curriculum, attend educational updates (at least yearly) and take opportunities to network and engage with fellow mentors.

Triennial review

Guidance for placement providers is also provided. Placement providers are responsible for holding and maintaining an up to date register of mentors, and this must be regularly reviewed to ensure that it has currency and is amended as necessary. All 'sign-off' mentors should also be annotated on the register of mentors. This database can then be utilized by HEI partners to assure themselves that there are sufficient mentors available to support students on placements and in practice learning. Also included is the expectation that placement providers will ensure that in order to remain active, a mentor will engage in a triennial (three yearly) review of their mentorship practice to provide assurance that mentors meet their regulatory body's professional standard in order to continue to practice as a mentor.

This triennial review should provide evidence that mentors and practice teachers have mentored two students (one for practice teachers) in the last three years; and have participated in an annual update which included the opportunity to engage with other mentors, and explored as a group the challenges to be encountered when assessing in challenging circumstances, and mapped their ongoing practice to the mentorship standards and ensured that they meet all these requirements to stay active on a 'live' register of mentors.

It is up to each placement provider to determine the exact nature of their triennial review process (NMC, 2008). The evidence for triennial review may take the form of a 'mentor portfolio' and this might not be dissimilar to a professional portfolio. Placement providers and HEIs have worked in partnership to create advice and local guidance for their mentors. One group of Practice Education Facilitators developed a mentor portfolio for use throughout their region. This document contains general information about mentorship and sign-off mentorship, Each domain and related outcomes has suggested forms of suitable evidence. There is also space to reflect on mentorship experience and evidence any 'sign-off' supervisory episodes.

Over to you

Find out how your employer manages this process. Is there a guideline or protocol? Have you started to map your own mentorship practice to the mentor standards?

The NMC undertakes quality assurance reviews of all NMC approved programmes of education through robust processes of approval and annual monitoring. This includes all programmes leading to registration or a record on the register, and programmes of preparation for individuals supporting learning and assessment in practice. Education institutions and their practice partners are monitored on an annual basis. As a result the strength of partnership working between these two stakeholders needs to visibly show that there is evidence of clear and transparent working and that they are able to demonstrate adherence to these standards when scrutinized by the NMC.

THE DOMAINS OF MENTORSHIP

The NMC (2008) identified competencies and outcomes under the following headings (Table 3.3) mapped to each stage: registrant; mentor; practice teacher and teacher

Table 3.3 Competencies and outcomes of the eight NMC domains	
Domain	**Nature of content**
Establishing effective working relationships	An understanding of the factors that influence a student integrating into the practice setting, the provision of ongoing and constructive support to facilitate transition from one learning environment to the next, building effective interpersonal relationships
Facilitation of learning	The selection of appropriate and individualized learning opportunities and strategies to integrate learning from practice and theory. Supporting students to reflect upon learning experiences

(Continued)

Table 3.3 Competencies and outcomes of the eight NMC domains (*Continued*)	
Domain	**Nature of content**
Assessment and accountability	Foster professional growth, personal development and accountability, demonstrate a breadth of understanding in regard to assessment,, provide constructive feedback and manage failing students – ultimately confirming that students have met or have not met the NMC competencies in practice. As a sign-off mentor they should confirm that students have met the NMC proficiencies
Evaluation of learning	Contribute to evaluation of student learning and assessment. Participate in self and peer evaluation to facilitate development
Creating an environment for learning	Identify learning needs and experiences that are appropriate to the student level of learning using a range of learning experiences. Identify aspects of the learning environment which could be enhanced and act as a resource to facilitate the development of others
Context of practice	Recognize the unique needs of the practice environment contributing to the development of an environment that supports achievement of the NMC standards of proficiency. Set and maintain professional boundaries as well as recognize the influence of the wider interprofessional team. Support students exploring new ways of working and the impact this may have.
Evidence-based practice	Identify areas for research and development, use local and national health frameworks to review and identify area for development. Develop new practitioners by advancing own professional knowledge to be able to meet changes in roles and care delivery. Disseminate research findings
Leadership	Provide practice leadership and expertise in application of knowledge and skills based on evidence. Lead education in practice with other partners. Manage the competing demands of practice and education, lead and contribute to evaluation of the effectiveness of learning and assessment in practice

NMC (2008)

The expectation at each stage increases exponentially and recognizes the changing role and developing skill set. For example in the 'Evaluation of learning' domain:

- stage 1 the registrant will be expected to contribute information related to those learning in practice, and about the nature of learning experiences, to enable those supporting students to make judgements on the quality of the learning environment

- stage 2 the mentor should contribute to the evaluation of student learning and assessment experiences and propose aspects for change that result from such evaluation

- stage 3 the practice teacher will design evaluation strategies to determine the effectiveness of practice and academic experience accessed by students at both registration level and those in education at a level beyond initial registration

● stage 4 the teacher determines and uses criteria for evaluating the effectiveness of learning environments, acting on the findings, with others to enhance quality. (Annexe 1, p. 52, NMC, 2008).

A self-assessment can be a useful starting point when planning or evidencing one's own mentorship practice. A strengths, weaknesses, threats and opportunities type of tool can be used, where the mentor maps out their view of each of these. One HEI uses a 'mentor wheel'. This is based on a life wheel (Harvey-Lloyd adapted from Whitworth *et al.,* 2008 and NMC, 2008) that has the domains of mentorship as spokes (see Figure 3.1). The mentor or practice teacher could then self assess, using the mentor standards, awarding a mark of one to ten in terms of 'satisfied' with that aspect of mentorship. Using the individual outcomes relevant for their particular stage and then actions can be devised in order to develop the two or three areas with the lowest score.

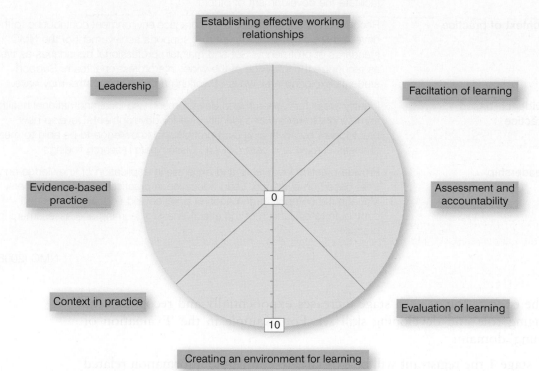

Figure 3.1   Using a life wheel to self assess with the NMC mentor domains
(adapted from Harvey-Lloyd and Whitworth *et al.,* 2008 and the NMC, 2008)

Over to you

Using the mentor wheel and the appropriate outcomes for your stage assess your development. Plan an action for one of the domains with the lowest score.

SIGN-OFF MENTORSHIP

An additional aspect to mentorship within stage 2 has also been identified, that of a 'sign-off' role. According to the NMC (2008, p. 6) 'The role of the sign-off mentor and/or practice teacher is to make judgments about whether a student has achieved the required standards of proficiency for safe and effective practice for entry to the NMC register.' This process is part of the overall assessment which makes up part of the NMC approval of the programme. The role is applied slightly differently across parts of the register. Students on NMC approved pre-registration midwifery education programmes, leading to registration on the midwives' part of the register, can only be supported and assessed by mentors who have met the additional sign-off criteria. However students on pre-registration nursing programmes only require sign-off mentors on the final placement. Sign-off mentors are also required for all students on specialist practice programmes leading to a recordable qualification on the nurses' part of the register (NMC, 2008).

Generally these 'sign-off' mentors are the more experienced ones who must demonstrate that they have met the sign-off mentor criteria in full and this includes being supervised for signing-off proficiency on three occasions by an appropriately qualified existing 'sign-off' mentor. A circular from the NMC published in March 2010 revised this part of the standard (NMC, 2010), so this now includes the possibility that the first two episodes of sign-off experience can be interactive simulations, however the final one must be with a final placement student (Aston and Hallam, 2011).

The NMC (2008) state that placement providers must ensure that a nurse or midwife identified as a sign-off mentor who assesses proficiency for a particular student at the end of a programme is:

- Annotated on the local register as a sign-off mentor or a practice teacher.
- Registered on the same part of the register.
- Working in the same field of practice as that in which the student intends to qualify.

Andrews *et al.* (p. 253, 2010) describe a sign-off mentor as a type of 'super mentor Glasper (2010b) reminds us that this is a challenging role that is regularly scrutinized by the NMC as part of their quality assurance activities.

Reflective activity

What do you think that the additional criteria for sign-off mentors might be?

You may have thought of skills like:

- much experience as a mentor
- effective practice as a nurse or midwife
- awareness of accountability and ethical consideration
- expertise in assessment and giving feedback.

To a degree, all of these things should be evident within any mentor, however in addition to these the sign-off mentor must demonstrate an understanding of the NMC registration requirements and the contribution that the sign-off makes to these.

There is no set time limit for nurses to become sign-off mentors. It may depend on the context of your practice learning environment, and the allocation of students or the nature of the learning experience offered. However, as stated previously, *all* midwifery mentors must be sign-off mentors and this should form a part of the mentor preparation programme and be supported by clear processes for the achievement of sign-off supervisory episodes.

Over to you

Look at the criteria for sign-off mentorship below and consider your own practice in relation to these.

- Clinical currency and capability in the field in which the student is being assessed.

- In possession of a working knowledge of current programme requirements, practice assessment strategies and relevant changes in education and practice for the student they are assessing.

- Able to demonstrate understanding of the NMC registration requirements and the contribution they make to the achievement of these requirements.

- An in-depth understanding of their accountability to the NMC for the decision they must make to pass or fail a student when assessing proficiency requirements at the end of a programme.

- Been supervised on at least three occasions for signing-off proficiency by an existing sign-off

- mentor.

- A working knowledge of current programme requirements, practice assessment strategies and relevant changes in education and practice for the student they are assessing. (NMC, 2008)

Do you meet this criteria? What would you need to do in addition to meet this?

PRACTICE TEACHERS

The NMC (2008) states that a practice teacher is a registrant who normally will have previously fulfilled the NMC requirements to become a mentor, and who has received further preparation to achieve the knowledge, skills and competence required to meet the NMC defined outcomes for a practice teacher.

All students undertaking a programme leading to registration as a specialist community public health nurse (SCPHN) are required to have a named practice teacher (NMC, 2008).

Health care professional

Practice teacher

It is a true privilege to be able to help develop the confidence of the 'students' as they progress, and to share their journey to becoming specialist practitioners and developing new skills and knowledge. I always put 'students' in inverted commas, as it's important to remember the wealth of skills and expertise these students bring with them to the programme, and it is always very much a two-way learning experience. The transition from nursing into specialist community public health practice can be disempowering to them for a while, and as a CPT it's important to try and lessen the impact. I always feel such a great sense of pride at graduation and recognize the honour of sharing with them a moment in time when all their hard work and dedication is being recognized, and they are now moving to a new phase in their professional careers.

With the increases in Health Visitor (SCPHN) students over the past year we have really worked hard to fully support student health visitors, and practice teachers have worked with the whole team to deliver a good practice learning environment. Trainee practice teachers must be supervised by an existing sign-off practice teacher on at least one occasion when they are signing-off proficiency of a SCPHN student at the end of their final placement.

The trainee practice teacher can be entered on the local register as a practice teacher on successful completion of the programme. After this they should then undertake a period of preceptorship supported by an existing sign-off practice teacher. What this entails is decided by the local placement provider. During this time further supervised sign-offs of SCPHN students should be undertaken.

Once the period of preceptorship is completed and the preceptor is satisfied that the preceptee is competent in signing-off proficiency the preceptee can be annotated as a sign-off practice teacher.

The practice teacher should continue to receive support from other experienced practice teachers when making final placement assessment decisions, until they have received the first triennial review and been identified as continuing to meet the criteria to be able to sign-off proficiently (NMC, 2008).

TEACHERS

The final stage in the standard is at Teacher level, and this is an NMC registrant who, following successful completion of an NMC approved teacher preparation programme, has achieved the knowledge, skills and competence required to meet the NMC defined outcomes of stage 4 of the developmental framework. The NMC teacher standard is mandatory for those nurses and midwives based in higher education who support learning and assessment in practice settings for students on NMC approved programmes.

KEY POINTS

● The NMC Standard to Support Learning and Assessment in Practice (2008) provides a single developmental framework for nurses.

● A sign-off mentor is a mentor who meets specific criteria identified in the standard.

All mentors are expected to map their practice to the NMC domains to ensure that they maintain currency and capability as a mentor.

CHALLENGES IN PRACTICE

It is evident that although there are clear benefits to undertaking the mentorship role, for example, as a result of providing support to students, mentors are more likely and required to keep up to date with their own skills and knowledge (Myall *et al.*, 2008). There are many challenges to be encountered when supporting practice learning and assessment. These originate from a variety of sources. The decisions that mentors make about a student's performance will have serious implications for the student and service user (Carr *et al.*, 2010) The efficacy of mentorship skills can be influenced by the opportunities given to practice them; particularly assessment and feedback, expertise and confidence as a practitioner, general support and facilitation by the clinical leader, demands of the care environment, the ability to prioritize and fundamentally the motivation to carry out the role. The literature reflects a variety of challenges in the mentorship and practice role which ranges from the impact of higher student numbers, how they are prepared for the role, whether there is any role confusion, whether they have ensured supernumery status, and managing competing demands with a willingness to undertake the role (McGowan, 2006; Bray and Nettleton, 2007; Rutowski, 2007; Omansky, 2010; Williamson *et al.*, 2010; Harries, 2011; Haydock *et al.*, 2011; Mead, 2011; Carr and Gidman, 2012).

We will explore some of these challenges in later chapters in more detail and consider aspects of how to feedback to students in an effective way here.

GIVING FEEDBACK

When a student is likeable and motivated but has achieved only poorly in terms of their clinical practice, it can be difficult to focus on the negative aspects of their practice; however this is required if they are to progress. Not only should mentors be equipped with the ability to undertake assessment, they also need to feel comfortable with giving negative feedback. Students should also learn to take feedback constructively. A learner needs to recognize feedback as feedback, although this can be informal in nature.

Reflective activity

Think about two occasions when you have been given negative feedback.

● The first one should be when you received negative feedback in a destructive manner. What did the person say to you? How did you feel as a result? What impact did the feedback have on your behaviour?

● Then think about a time when you received negative feedback in a more constructive manner. What did the person say to you? How did you feel as a result? What impact did the feedback have on your behaviour?

● What does this suggest to you about giving feedback to students on their practice working?

Giving students feedback means letting them know how they are performing, in a timely and ongoing way. Feedback may be formal or informal. Formal feedback is planned as part of the assessment and occurs episodically, usually covering the specific learning outcomes to be achieved. Informal feedback should be given on a daily basis in relation to specific events related to patient care. Giving negative feedback can be hard to do, but a positive critique starts when the student is asked to speak first. It is important that you own your feedback by saying 'I think'/ I have seen – or similar. It is good to remember that criticism only improves performance when: it is timely and constructive:

● it is given in an appropriate setting
● it is given with genuine liking for the person
● you have sought the other person's explanation
● it is related to specific instances
● it focuses on the behaviours rather than the person
● you describe the behaviour rather than judge it
● you look beneath the surface
● you look for alternative ways forward
● you allow opportunity for reflection.

Learners require constructive and informative feedback as soon as possible after the practice event if the feedback is to be meaningful, and they need to be given the opportunity to develop self-assessment and reflective skills.

Over to you

Read the following excerpt from a mentor–mentee midway review meeting. If you were advising the student or the practitioner what would you suggest to help improve the giving and receiving of feedback in this situation?

Mentor: I wanted to mention today, because I have been thinking for a while, that your communication with patients is not as good as it could be.

Mentee: What's the matter with it?

Mentor: Well (pause), sometimes you're a bit short in your communication style. You say what you need to get across to patients but you aren't very chatty or conversational.

Mentee: It's really busy in here and I've been working really hard. So there hasn't been time to chat.

Mentor: I know it is busy, but Angela – the other student in your group – manages to chat whilst she is delivering her care.

Mentee: Angela was a nursing assistant before she came on the course, so she's more used to working on a ward.

For feedback to be effective a mentor needs to be plain speaking and specific about the action or behaviour that is being referred to. Therefore, a descriptive and detailed example can be helpful. The focus should be on the actions or behaviours, not on the individual. There should be a balance, praising good work as well as pointing out areas that require improvement, as feedback given in this way is more likely be accepted. So in the 'Over to you' excerpt, acknowledging the hard work of the student would have been appropriate. Offering constructive suggestions of ways to improve the situation is also helpful. It would have been better to have focused on what the student could do to improve rather than focusing on comparison to another learner.

TOP TIPS

- Let the student/learner speak first
- Begin with the good points
- Be specific rather than general (limit what you cover)
- Plan a solution for each problem
- Show interest, respect and involvement

- Be constructive (describe the problem that exists)
- Deal with one point at a time (give the learner time to think)
- Offer a critique of the act rather than the individual
- Do not hyperbolize (try not to use terms such as 'never', 'always')
- Do not joke
- Do not compare
- Take account of the receiver's needs
- Check that the receiver has understood
- Be productive (end on a positive note) and support for improvement

Receiving negative feedback

In the first moments when the student realizes that they are receiving criticism, they are likely to react as anyone would: their heart beats faster and their skin temperature goes down because they feel under attack, and instinctually they will focus on that feeling, making it more intense. This can lead to the student feeling like withdrawing or retaliating. On receiving negative feedback, the recipient's first instinct may be to look for ways in which they themselves can be viewed as right, and the momentum of defensive emotions builds fast as they focus mentally on the 'right' things that they are doing. There can also be a tendency to obsess about the thoughtless and 'wrong' things that the other person, the mentor, is viewed as doing. This can lead to a rigid, defensive and non-listening stance. So it is helpful if the student, when receiving negative feedback, tries to think about the good points of the mentor. They are then more likely to be generous and react calmly towards the mentor, which increases the possibility that the meeting outcome will be more positive and there will also be opportunities to look at the areas of 'good' practice in a balanced way.

Steps in responding to negative feedback

Step one: Acknowledge

- Acknowledge that you heard the mentor: for example, nod your head and pause, allowing you time to think about this and to cool down. Do not disagree or counter-attack, instead make a comment such as 'I understand you have a concern...'

Step two: Ask for more

- Ask for more information so that the focus is on the issue, not the feelings or personalities. Focus – mentally and/or verbally – on the aspects of the mentor that you respect.

Step three: Add your own

● If you believe the comments are accurate, acknowledge this and add your own. Then say what you plan to do differently to respond to the negative feedback; the mentor is then likely to add their actions to help towards improved practice. If you disagree with the feedback comments, ask for permission to give your reasons why, and then a constructive discussion regarding this issue can occur.

In some situations, students can feel that feedback is not very forth-coming, and if this is the case they should request it. However, when seeking feedback you need to be aware that you might hear criticism as well as praise. Try to divorce the content of the feedback from the giver and recognize that it has the potential to transform your personal and professional development.

Student

Student nurse

When I was on one ward the mentor gave me feedback that I was not getting involved in aspects of practice which I needed to develop at my stage of training. For example, offering to assist with medication rounds. I felt annoyed at first because I thought that as the ward was busy, I had been right to focus on the essential patient care rather than appearing to focus on just getting certain competencies signed off. However, when we went on to discuss this further I realized that I had been avoiding offering to assist with medication rounds as I felt that my pharmacology knowledge was not at the same level as the other students in my group and it had started to become a hidden worry. By the end of the placement, when we had worked on my confidence in this area, I valued my mentor for taking the time to work with me on this and to give me the feedback in time to allow me to act on it.

Most health care courses are now continuously assessed in practice throughout each placement. Practice assessment of clinical competence is extremely important, but confusion can be created by the multiplicity of terms used within practice-based assessment, such as competencies, learning outcomes and capability. According to McMullan *et al.* (2003) competence and competencies are job related and demonstrated through performance, whereas competency and competencies are person orientated and encompass individual characteristics and qualities. If practitioners base their assessment of practice on overall competency rather than reviewing specific competencies, their judgement is more likely to be subjective and difficult to demonstrate.

The practice assessment tools supplied by higher education institutes can make it difficult for mentors to recognize the essential elements of practice when assessing, but familiarity with the assessment tool makes this less problematic. Mentors and clinical educators/lecturers need to work together in the development and use of practice assessment tools to increase the likelihood of as objective a judgement as possible. In order to adequately gauge the student's knowledge, skills and attitudes, the assessment process and methodology need to be clear and understood by the mentor.

A new mentor may be anxious because they do not want to get their assessment wrong and jeopardize an individual's professional career, so they may give the student the 'benefit of the doubt' when their practice work appears to be a borderline pass/fail. It has been found that mentors who lack mentorship experience or confidence are reluctant to give a student a fail grade (Duffy, 2004).

SUPPORTING UNDERACHIEVING LEARNERS

Much discussion has been given to supporting underachieving students. This remains one of the most pivotal areas of mentorship practice. Gopee (2008) says that mentoring practices need to be congruent with ethical and legal aspects of patient care with the accountability for assessment decisions being key.

Duffy's (2004) seminal research around why mentors 'fail to fail' students discovered that students are passing clinical assessments even when there are doubts about their competency. Mentors were found unwilling to document their concerns, lecturers identifying that weak students continued to progress. Failing a student was considered very difficult, demanding and emotional as well as affected by practical issues.

With appropriate support and reflection on the experience, future practice of the mentor can be enhanced. When utilizing a reflective model to think about mentorship, Carr et al. (2010) found unexpectedly that the challenges encountered and the personal impact of these could be felt months after the events linked to failing students had happened. When considering efficacy and mentorship practice related to supporting under-achieving students, it could be argued that improved practice will result in fewer referrals, with students who require help getting this, which allows them to succeed. Andrews et al. (2010) add to the debate proposing that although the notion of sign-off mentors is to protect the public and provide extra support at the end of a programme it could be viewed as counter-productive as it would be more beneficial to address performance issues at an earlier stage. Without doubt mentoring a student who is failing can be very challenging for a mentor. Jervis and Tilki (2011) concur with earlier reports that it can be emotionally demanding, stressful and possibly threatening for the mentor and in our experience a good deal of tenacity and commitment is required. Casey and Clark (2011) cite a reluctance to fail students early in a programme as a recurrent theme in the literature, suggesting that mentors may assume that improvement will occur over time.

In some cases it is necessary for a mentor to refer or fail a student because they do not meet the necessary competencies. When this does happen, the mentor should identify this issue as early as possible to the student; it is also important that the mentor contacts the higher education institute link or local practice education contact. This means that support is mobilized for both the student and the mentor. The action plan that is then devised is understood by all involved, and there may be an opportunity for another assessor to add their assessment to the mentor's. Further guidance around the development of an action plan to support an underachieving learner can be found as a bonus feature in the online resource that accompanies this chapter. Records must be kept of all discussions, action plans and any observations of practice undertaken during this period of support for a potentially failing student. Walsh (2010, p. 184) has a golden rule 'Get to know your students and the level they are at early on'. This is crucial as timely intervention is essential. It can be useful to utilize a flow chart which ensures that due process is followed, this is often developed to meet local resource and need, but essentially offers similar guidance (see Figure 3.2 on the next page).

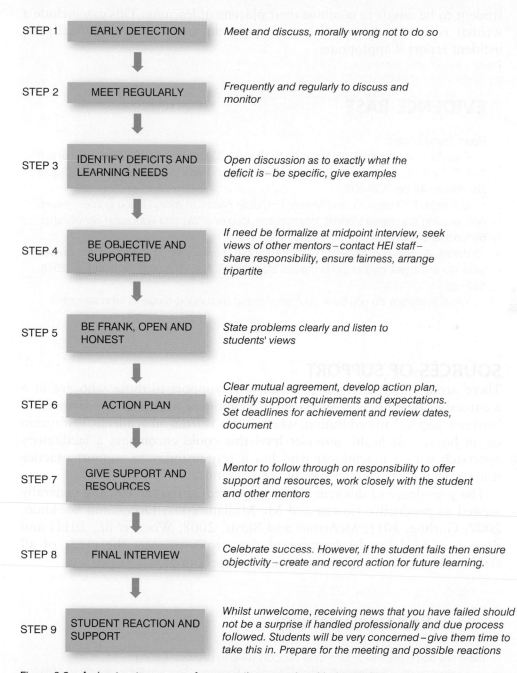

STEP 1	EARLY DETECTION	*Meet and discuss, morally wrong not to do so*
STEP 2	MEET REGULARLY	*Frequently and regularly to discuss and monitor*
STEP 3	IDENTIFY DEFICITS AND LEARNING NEEDS	*Open discussion as to exactly what the deficit is – be specific, give examples*
STEP 4	BE OBJECTIVE AND SUPPORTED	*If need be formalize at midpoint interview, seek views of other mentors – contact HEI staff – share responsibility, ensure fairness, arrange tripartite*
STEP 5	BE FRANK, OPEN AND HONEST	*State problems clearly and listen to students' views*
STEP 6	ACTION PLAN	*Clear mutual agreement, develop action plan, identify support requirements and expectations. Set deadlines for achievement and review dates, document*
STEP 7	GIVE SUPPORT AND RESOURCES	*Mentor to follow through on responsibility to offer support and resources, work closely with the student and other mentors*
STEP 8	FINAL INTERVIEW	*Celebrate success. However, if the student fails then ensure objectivity – create and record action for future learning.*
STEP 9	STUDENT REACTION AND SUPPORT	*Whilst unwelcome, receiving news that you have failed should not be a surprise if handled professionally and due process followed. Students will be very concerned – give them time to take this in. Prepare for the meeting and possible reactions*

Figure 3.2   A step by step process for supporting an underachieving student
(adapted from Walsh, 2010)

More rarely, a mentor may meet a situation where a student is unsafe in practice. This should be discussed straight away with the senior clinical lead in the practice area and the educational link from the higher education institute. It is crucial that the mentor records their reasons for deeming the student to be unsafe to continue their placement learning. This can include a written report in the practice assessment document and additionally an incident report if appropriate.

EVIDENCE BASE

Read these articles:

Cleland, J. A., Knight, L. V., Rees, C. E., Tracey, S., Bond, C. M. (2008) Is it me or is it them? Factors that influence the passing of underperforming students. *Medical Education.* **42** pp. 800–809.

Luhanga, F., Yonge, O. and Myrick, F. (2008) Failure to assign failing grades: Issues with grading the unsafe student. *International Journal of Nursing Education Scholarship.* **5**(1) article 8 pp. 1–14.

Jervis, A. and Tilki, M. (2011) Why are nurse mentors failing to fail student nurses who do not meet clinical performance standards? *British Journal of Nursing.* **20**(9): 582–587.

What strategies do you think you can develop to support students who struggle?

SOURCES OF SUPPORT

There are a variety of roles that can offer support to those who are in a mentorship type of role. An essential component of this is the partnership between 'service' and education, whether this is from an academic institution or 'in house'. At health provider level this could encompass a facilitatory approach with a practitioner who has a responsibility to support practice learner, to the link lecturer role of the academic.

The prevalence of different roles is reported across the UK and generally viewed as productive (Jowett and Mc Mullan, 2007; Elcock and Sookhoo, 2007; Gurling, 2011; McArthur and Burns, 2008; Wood *et al.,* 2011) and there is a need for development of these roles to meet the needs of all stakeholders and to implement these roles appropriately.

Reflective activity

Here are some titles for educational support roles in practice settings:

Clinical Practice Facilitator; Practice Education Facilitator; Practice Educator; Clinical Placement Facilitator; Learning Community Education Advisors; Link Mentor; Link Lecturer.

Identify if any of these are available in your practice setting.

Think of the roles you have locally. Who could offer you support in your role as a mentor?

How would you make contact with these individuals?

Who could advise you in the first instance?

In this chapter we have explored professional mentorship, and whilst the content has referred to the NMC requirements for nurses and midwives, as highlighted previously many of the skills and qualities required and challenges encountered will be similar throughout the health care related professions.

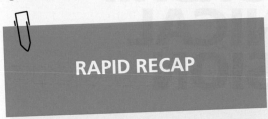

RAPID RECAP

Check your progress so far by working through each of the following questions.

1 What are the main responsibilities of a mentor?

2 Which students require a sign-off mentor?

3 How should a mentor handle a situation where a student is performing poorly and is at risk of failing their practice assessment in the placement?

4 What is a triennial review?

If you have difficulty with any of these questions, read through the section again to refresh your understanding before moving on.

CHAPTER 4
PRECEPTORSHIP AND CLINICAL SUPERVISION

LEARNING OBJECTIVES

By the end of this chapter you should be able to:

● define the main facilitator roles that support the learning of registered practitioners within practice

● appreciate the importance of preceptorship and clinical supervision

● explore methods of enhancing clinical skills development and assessment

● value interpersonal communication and relationship building in allowing the effective giving and receiving of feedback.

Bonus features for this chapter available on the book's website

INTRODUCTION

An important stage in learning through practice occurs at the point of practitioner qualification and is termed the preceptorship period; this is when the newly qualified practitioner will require support by a competent role model in making the transition from student to competent practitioner. As professionals settle into their qualified practice, many professions require continued formal clinical supervision, and this is looked at later in the chapter.

Both of these activities support practice development and the provision of services as a whole. They are concerned with enabling staff to be safe and effective practitioners.

UNDERPINNING INFLUENCES

In order to deliver the best possible service, it seems reasonable that those who do so should be functioning at an optimal level. In health and social care, whether it be in an NHS Trust or in an independent third sector organization, we all work in teams, and every individual has an important contribution to make to the success of care (DoH, 2008, *A High Quality Workforce*). The ethos of lifelong learning is essential to everyday practice. In 2001 in 'Working together – Learning together' the Secretary for State said that:

> *Lifelong learning is about growth and opportunity, about making sure that our staff, the teams and organizations they relate to, and work in, can acquire new knowledge and skills, both to realize their potential and to help shape and change things for the better.*
>
> DoH, 2001, p. i

This is as relevant today as it was then and it is still evident in every staff member's responsibility and supported by professional codes. The NHS constitution says that patients:

> *Have **the right** to be treated with a professional standard of care, by appropriately qualified and experienced staff.*
>
> DoH, 2012, p. 6

In addition to this the NHS is committed to provide all staff with personal development and access to appropriate training for their jobs, and staff are expected to take up any opportunities afforded to them (DoH, 2012).

Therefore a conscious focused attempt to develop oneself is absolutely necessary and in the best interests of all stakeholders. This can be striving to attain Maslow's self-actualization through personal and professional growth as a result of clinical supervision, or meeting the lower order needs of safety and security when embarking on your career as a registered practitioner starting that first job.

ESSENTIAL COMPONENTS

Preceptorship

A preceptor is a person who teaches, counsels, inspires, serves as a role model and supports the growth and development of an individual (novice practitioner) for a fixed and limited amount of time with the specific purpose of

Preceptorship involves a supportive one-to-one teaching and learning relationship between an experienced and competent role model and a newly qualified practitioner; it is for a specified time period and is to help the practitioner to adjust to their new professional role

assisting them into their new role. The term was first used within nursing in America in the 1970s to identify an experienced qualified nurse who, working in partnership with a newly qualified member of the nursing profession, assists the latter to adapt to their new role in a fixed period post-qualification (Morton-Cooper and Palmer, 1993). The preceptorship period within nursing is usually around four–six months.

Being a preceptor can be fulfilling and rewarding. The main difference between being a mentor and a preceptor is that the latter is facilitating a peer, requiring an 'enabling' relationship. Morton-Cooper and Palmer (1993) suggest that an enabler is:

- **comfortable** with themselves and their abilities
- **accessible** and able to create mutual respect
- **responsive** to others needs
- **easy to trust.**

The preceptor's knowledge of the organization, team and clinical practice is seen as invaluable to the newly qualified practitioner, although the preceptee, as a registered practitioner, remains accountable for their actions. Preceptorship of an individual is primarily concerned with easing the transition from learner to practitioner, thereby limiting the damage of 'reality shock' (Kramer, 1974), 'Reality shock' occurs when the practitioner realizes the enormity of staying within one clinical setting and taking on the responsibilities of a qualified practitioner. Through the preceptor's facilitation, supervision and acting as a role model, the newly qualified practitioner is able to achieve an effective transition from being a student.

EVIDENCE BASE

Read: DoH (2010a) *Preceptorship Framework for Newly Registered Nurses, Midwives and Allied Heath Professionals*. DoH, London.

In a study exploring the first year of practice, Tryssenar and Perkins (2001) found four stages were identified: transition, euphoria and angst, reality of practice and adaptation. Recognizing the stages of development within the first year of qualified practice can help those who are supporting practitioners. As well as enhancing the clinical performance and skills development of a new practitioner, the preceptorship period should help in the socializing of new team members into a practice community. It is argued that offering a formal, supportive preceptorship relationship increases staff retention, reduces stress and helps to bridge the period between the students' receiving mentorship and their progressing towards clinical supervision (Myrick and Yonge, 2001).

There can be great variations between different preceptors, preceptees, clinical settings and professional groups in their understanding and implementation of preceptorship. Although there is structured entry to many health care professions following initial qualification, the professions may well not define this as preceptorship, terming it an extension of clinical supervision.

If the needs of the preceptor, preceptee and organization are to be met (see Figure 4.1), it is helpful if this is approached in a structured way.

The needs of a newly qualified practitioner are usually broadly based around:

- reviewing what they have achieved to date
- understanding what is expected of them
- adapting to their new role and developing new clinical skills
- continuing to learn and develop in their clinical practice
- performing effectively in their patient care
- feeling valued as part of a team.

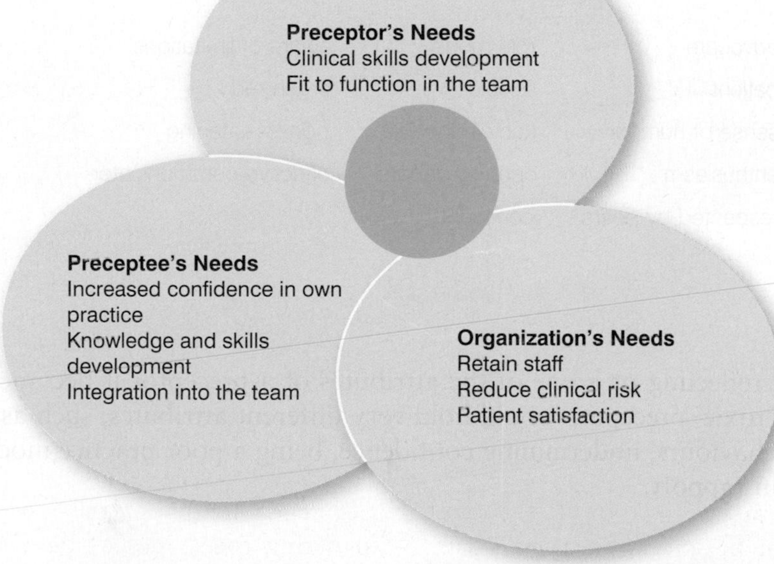

Preceptor's Needs
Clinical skills development
Fit to function in the team

Preceptee's Needs
Increased confidence in own practice
Knowledge and skills development
Integration into the team

Organization's Needs
Retain staff
Reduce clinical risk
Patient satisfaction

Figure 4.1   Needs to be addressed within a preceptorship learning contract

Staff in the clinical setting need to be involved in the development of a structured programme of preceptorship, including planning the preceptorship programme, involvement in education and awareness sessions, and evaluating the preceptorship programme. The aim should be that all those involved identify the benefits of a structured approach and that these benefits are realized.

Key areas to formalize for preceptorship in a clinical setting

- The role of the preceptor, the relationship of the preceptor and preceptee within a preceptorship programme
- Who requires preceptorship – newly qualified staff, those returning from breaks in service and those returning after working for a significant time in a very different speciality
- The format for guidelines/documentation of the preceptorship period
- Practical issues, training and support resources available
- Linkage to current arrangements – informal structures for support

Reflective activity

Have you got what it takes to be a preceptor? Look at the attributes identified below and reflect on those you currently possess, those you would like to work on and add any others that you think are also important.

advocate	role model	aware of limitations
patient	flexible	organized
sense of humour	knowledgeable	non-threatening
enthusiasm	open to debate	effective communicator
respected by peers	confident	

When reflecting on some of the attributes of a preceptor it becomes clear that the 'toxic' preceptor would hold very different attributes, such as threatening behaviours, undermining confidence, being a poor practice model and lacking in rapport.

KEY POINTS

- The relationship between the preceptor and preceptee is that of a peer
- The preceptee remains accountable for actions and practice
- The initial transitional period can be challenging for the preceptee

Preceptorship approaches and models

With the advent of the Agenda for Change payscale (2004) practitioners working in the NHS should be offered a preceptorship period in the first year (NHS Employers, 2012). The Department of Health (DoH) published a Preceptorship Framework for Newly Registered Nurses, Midwives and Allied Health Professionals which details best practice, including topics such as the benefits and implementation of preceptorship (2010a). According to this document, preceptorship should be individualized and meet the needs of the local context. The indicative content can drawn from areas shown in Figure 4.2. 'Flying start NHS' a web based resource, is useful and informative in regard to preceptorship.

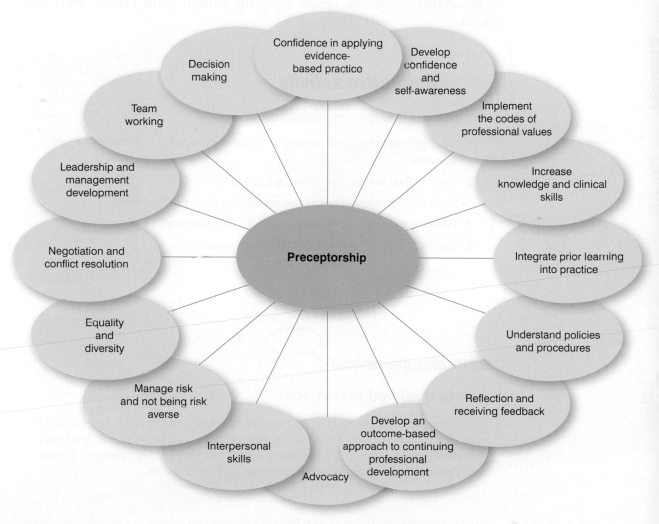

Figure 4.2 Indicative content of preceptorship programmes, (DoH, 2010, public domain)

Over to you

Many organizations have a policy or guideline on preceptorship, see if you can find your local information. Were you familiar with the contents?

Preceptor as a role model

One of the attributes you reflected on in the last activity was the preceptor as role model. Role modelling involves studying the behavioural patterns of sound professional practitioners, and it could be argued that those selected to be preceptors should be people who, the clinical team believe, meet this criteria.

Reflective activity

Reflect on your answers to the following questions.

1 What are the behavioural patterns of successful practitioners in the area in which you work?

2 How do they achieve their client-care results?

3 What do they do that is more successful than other practitioners?

4 What are the skills and qualities that make the difference?

5 Are these practitioners best placed to be preceptors?

Health care professional

Newly qualified practitioner

I really enjoyed my course and looked forward to finishing but now I'm worried about what people expect of me. I'm the same person today as I was yesterday but now I have a qualified nurse's uniform. Not everybody knows that I'm new. My preceptor is really nice, I'm just not sure how we're going to meet and set goals yet.

Working with a role model does not mean simply replicating what they do: it involves explaining why and how one can achieve similar outcomes and requires 'thinking', as well as 'doing' in a similar way to a practitioner who is at the peak of their practice. There are three aspects to the modelling process. For instance, if a new practitioner wishes to improve their assessment skills, they will initially watch the preceptor whilst they assess a patient. During this observation, the preceptee imagines themselves doing this assessment, focusing on behaviours (what is done), internal thinking (how they do it) and the supporting assumptions, beliefs and knowledge (why they do it in that way). The 'what' is understood by direct observation, but the preceptee will only understand the 'how' and 'why' by asking questions. Having the opportunity to work alongside a 'role model' can help to increase clinical performance; however, each person brings their own unique resources and personality to a situation so this is only one strategy to help the novice practitioner.

As the preceptee is a qualified practitioner, it is important to acknowledge their individual accountability and that the preceptee must play an active part in their personal development. Preceptor qualities and skills identified as essential are leadership and communication skills, decision-making ability and an interest in professional growth. A preceptor should be willing to teach and have flexibility in providing an individualized learning experience. Support and advice should be available to preceptors to help them develop in their crucial role, and clinical supervision is an ideal forum for this. Like the mentor, the preceptor has two potentially conflicting roles – confidante and assessor – and this difficulty is further compounded by peer-evaluating another health care professional's work. Unfortunately the preceptorship period can sometimes be poorly structured; Gerrish (2000) found that some new practitioners were left to cope with little formal support.

Ground rules

Agreeing a set of ground rules for the preceptorship period can help 'set the scene' for an appropriate relationship. Ground rules are an agreed set of standards that allow meaningful dialogue to proceed with the aim of minimizing conflict and increasing the effectiveness of the pair/group. To be effective, the rules must be agreed upon by everyone involved beforehand. Any deviation in practice away from the agreed ground rules should be reviewed by those involved. Ground rules make each role and the expectations of this role clear. This involves setting up an individual learning contract and objectives based on the job description, competencies and the knowledge and skills profile for the position. The preceptorship documentation should provide the basis for an initial Individual Performance Review (IPR) or appraisal process and the development of a further personal development plan. For further detail on how to get the most out of learning contracts, refer to Chapter 5.

Preceptorship programme

During the first week of the preceptorship period, the preceptor meets with the preceptee and orientates the new practitioner to the clinical team, documentation, equipment and the communication channels in use. Any health and safety issues must also be discussed early on. Subsequent meetings are likely to focus on progress towards the learning objectives set up in the learning contract and any reflections on clinical working recorded by the new practitioner in their learning diary. Reflecting on practice in a diary can allow a practitioner to keep a record of their progress during this important time of transition and to identify any issues they want to address with their preceptor; this can lead to a re-negotiation of the learning contract. In addition to one-to-one meetings with a preceptor, it can be supportive and informative if a newly qualified staff member can continue to meet with their peer group, as this adds another dimension to their support structures at this stressful, transitional time.

KEY POINTS

Preceptorship programmes need:

- Flexibility in the programme to meet individual needs, with allowance for a variable time scale to achieve this.

- Education and support for preceptors and preceptees so that each takes an active role in the process; case scenarios are useful adjuncts to this.

- A framework or guidelines for the preceptorship period, based on the practitioner competencies and Foundation Knowledge and Skills Framework (KSF) outline (fast-track incremental progression is linked to successful achievement of preceptorship).

- Development of a learning package for preceptors, including definition, aims and objectives of preceptorship (within the NHS), role and responsibilities, training to be attended.

- A formal meeting and review of preceptorship learning at approximately one-month, three-month and six-month periods, with the intention that the preceptorship period will normally be completed at the final review meeting.

- In nursing and midwifery, a registered first-level practitioner who is already a 'sign-off' mentor, with at least 12 months' post-registration experience within the clinical setting to undertake the role (NMC, 2008).

- Preceptors with a willingness to share their skills, knowledge and attitude towards their work, and the ability to give feedback/evaluations on progress.

Clinical supervision

Clinical supervision is a formal process between a skilled supervisor and supervisee that enables a professional to reflect on and assume responsibility for their practice, and develop skills, knowledge and understanding of their practice whilst feeling supported. It is advocated for all clinical practitioners as it enhances consumer protection and safety of care in increasingly complex clinical situations.

Where possible, a clinical supervisor should observe a supervisee working; there should also be regular meetings. These meetings can be in a small group or just between the two individuals, and the main content is a review of recent working and the formulation of an action plan for future professional learning. The participants reflect on clinical experiences together, considering alternative ways of tackling issues, and discuss what they have learnt from the clinical experiences. They then agree how this will be applied and evidenced in the work setting in the near future.

Given the broad nature of clinical supervision, there is scope for overlap and confusion with other managerial and development activities. Supervision can take place in different formats, including clinical, managerial and training supervision. Clinical supervision enables a focus on professional competencies and high standards of the delivery of care. Managerial supervision is concerned with the monitoring of work commissioned by an organization. Training supervision is related to the acquisition of specific skills and competencies, and accountability is often linked to an educational establishment. The learning element of clinical supervision means that there is possible confusion between clinical supervision as outlined here and mentoring students. Clinical supervision is about a professional partnership, not an expert-to-novice relationship, although many of the skills and qualities required for mentorship are also required to deliver effective clinical supervision. For instance, support is offered both verbally and non-verbally (showing concern, giving praise, listening, providing space, offering guidance and advice, showing humour and giving time).

Reflective activity

Think about the situation where the clinical supervisor is also the line manager. Do you think confidentiality may be harder to maintain, or that it would be more difficult to establish the same levels of trust and openness?

Think about the clinical supervision in your current practice setting: what anxieties or concerns do you have about this? What possible problems have you had to contend with?

Clinical supervision should not be viewed as replacing other forms of staff support such as counselling services; however, it can make a contribution to reducing the negative outcomes of professional stress (Williamson and Dodds, 1999). Clinical supervision is an important way of developing professional skills and attributes, and this professional relationship between two qualified practitioners is ideally separate from any management structure. The focus is on individual reflection on practice, understanding and interpreting accurately the care provided, with the outcome being the identification of development needs. The concept of the reflective practitioner has implications for clinical supervision on two levels – the process requires reflection on real experiences from practice, and the clinical supervision process should help develop the ability to reflect critically on practice. Supervision can take place before or after an event and can be either planned or *ad hoc*.

Four main themes in clinical supervision

- A formal arrangement
- Interactive partnership
- Reflection on practice
- Professional and personal development

The United Kingdom Central Council for Nursing, Midwifery and Health Visiting (1996) produced a position statement on clinical supervision for nurses and health visitors and this has been endorsed by the Nursing and Midwifery Council. The six key principles of this position statement are:

1 Clinical supervision supports practice, enabling practitioners to maintain and promote standards of care.

2 Clinical supervision is a practice-focused professional relationship involving a practitioner reflecting on practice guided by a skilled supervisor.

3 Practitioners and managers should develop their own approach to clinical supervision, taking into account local circumstances. Ground rules should be agreed so that practitioners and supervisors are aware of what is involved and can trust in the confidentiality of clinical supervision.

4 Every practitioner should have access to clinical supervision, and a supervisor should supervise a realistic number of practitioners.

5 Preparation for supervisors can be delivered 'in house' or through external education programmes, but the importance of clinical supervision should be stressed in both pre- and post-registration educational programmes.

6 Evaluation and research regarding clinical supervision are needed to assess how it influences care, practice standards and the service delivered.

Although not a statutory requirement for nurses or health visitors, clinical supervision is a statutory function for midwives, as described in the Midwives Rules and Standards (NMC, 2004b). This states that clinical supervision is considered as integral to midwifery practice and that a midwifery supervisor should have no more than 15 midwives to supervise. Clinical supervision is also integral to many other health professions: for example, clinical psychologists, counsellors, occupational therapists, physiotherapists, dieticians and social workers have already developed systems of supervision.

Benefits of clinical supervision

Changes in clinical practice, organizational roles and structures, and patient expectations continue to create new challenges for health care professionals. Whilst these new challenges may in some cases offer exciting opportunities, they also place increasing demands on the practitioners who must respond. There has, therefore, been a movement in all health care professions towards clinical supervision as a tool to combat stress, maintain standards and enhance personal and professional development. There has been growing evidence of increased stress and, in some instances, burnout, resulting from the conflict between the care needs of clients and the demands of the organization.

> **Burnout**
> Burnout is different from stress, as it causes people who have previously been highly committed to their work to become disillusioned and to lose motivation and interest.
> Sufferers of burnout complain of physical, emotional and mental exhaustion which lead to a sense of reduced personal achievement and a lack of concern for patients.

EVIDENCE BASE

In 2011 30 per cent of NHS staff overall reported that they had experienced work-related stress (DoH, 2012b).

Take a look at the following journal articles:

- Davey et al. (2009) Predictors of nurse absenteeism in hospitals: a systematic review. *Journal of Nursing Management,* **17**: 312–330.

- Hallsten et al. (2011) Job burnout and job wornout as risk factors for long-term sickness absence. *Work,* **38**: 181–192.

Do you think there could be evidence of this within a health care setting you have had experience of?

The pace of change has also made it increasingly difficult for individual professionals to keep up to date with new developments and the evidence about the effectiveness and appropriateness of particular interventions or therapies. The combination of these issues can raise concern in relation to standards.

There are potential benefits for a health professional receiving clinical supervision, for the clinical supervisor, the supervisee, for the organization in which they work, and for patients and clients.

Health care professional

Clinical supervisee

At first it was quite challenging being involved in group clinical supervision, it took some time to build up trust. But it definitely helped me to develop my practice and face up to some things that I knew I had struggled with before. If I chose to discuss it in the session then I knew that I would have to do something about it. I think that I made myself do this, I wasn't under pressure but did feel challenged by my colleagues. They were very supportive. When we had been going for a while I used to think to myself 'what would they say to me?' if I encountered something which I needed to tackle. As it was group supervision we learnt to question each other and share this experience.

Reflective activity

To identify the potential benefits of clinical supervision, think about the learning, supportive and quality aspects of clinical supervision and then note down the benefits for each of the following:

● the individual professional receiving clinical supervision

● the clinical supervisor

● the organization

● patients/clients/service users.

Many researchers have tried to determine the benefits in learning and support that health care professionals' gain through clinical supervision. In some cases, researchers have evaluated the use of a particular clinical supervision model: in most instances, they found that supervisors and supervisees felt generally positive about the experience of supervision. When dissatisfaction with clinical supervision is expressed, it tends to relate to supervision taking time away from direct patient care, with nurses feeling guilty for leaving colleagues to work while they receive supervision. Butterworth *et al.* (1997) found that participant benefits included the availability of time to reflect on and learn from practice, the development of self-esteem, feeling supported by peers, taking responsibility for their own practice, and feeling more honest, relaxed, enthusiastic and less competitive. However, like many researchers, Butterworth *et al.* also acknowledge that it is harder to attribute improvements in patient care directly to clinical supervision. Edwards *et al.* (2006) explored how clinical supervision might affect the levels of 'burnout' in community mental health nurses and concluded that effective clinical supervision could lower levels.

Practical arrangements for clinical supervision

Clinical supervision contracts are usually recommended as this helps ensure clarity of roles and responsibilities, and is likely to formalize the need to undertake adequate preparation. Supervision contracts help to:

● prepare for a situation where supervisee and supervisor have different expectations of supervision with a subsequent reduction in the effectiveness of the supervisory relationship

● negotiate mutual expectations at the formative stages of supervision to help avoid problems later in supervision

● ensure working in supervision is structured, collaborative and begins to establish a pattern of attention in supervision to the process, content and relationship in order to be reflexive

- establish professional boundaries through making explicit the developmental, professional and legal functions of supervision
- create an underpinning foundation so that both supervisee and supervisor feel safe and supported.

Decisions to be made in agreeing the clinical supervision contract include:

- the type of supervision offered e.g. peer, one to one
- ground rules and policy regarding confidentiality
- suitability of the type of supervision to the supervisee's current needs
- the clinical supervision model and techniques that will be used
- the emphasis of the supervision, e.g. process, content and relationship
- practical considerations, e.g. meeting room, frequency, duration, note taking
- goals, aims and objectives of clinical supervision and the need to make them SMART (Specific, Measurable, Attainable, Relevant and Time limited)
- the rights and responsibilities of both the supervisee and supervisor
- how the effectiveness of supervision will be measured/evaluated
- how any problems will be handled from both the supervisee's and supervisor's perspectives
- how issues that are outside the competence of the supervisor will be handled
- how poor or incompetent practice will be addressed from both a supervisee and supervisor perspective
- the process of review and renegotiations of the supervision contract.

Ground rules for clinical supervision

Taking into account the need to challenge blocks in practice and to find time within a busy clinical schedule to meet, it becomes clear that it is necessary for those involved in the supervision process to agree 'ground rules' at the start.

Ground rules for supervision commonly cover confidentiality, complying with codes of professional conduct and treating each other with respect.

Over to you

If you are already involved in clinical supervision (either giving or receiving), review your ground rules and determine whether these need updating or revising in the light of what you have learnt from this chapter.

If you are not in a supervisory relationship construct at least four rules that you would like to see in a set of ground rules for your future supervision.

When, where and how long the supervisee and supervisor will meet needs to be planned and rostered into clinical working arrangements. It is common to meet from once a month to every six weeks; one-to-one supervision is likely to require at least 45 minutes to one hour; group supervision will require longer (but no more than two hours). A time needs to be identified that suits everyone; it should be when people are less likely to be called upon or interrupted. An appropriate place needs to be arranged where supervisory discussions can go ahead in confidence without risk of being disturbed or overheard. Contact details should be updated regularly in case any arrangements need modifying.

Within sessions it is vital to manage time, sticking to agreed timings for each session, monitoring how long is spent on each topic, and highlighting potential risks before they occur. Participants in the supervision session will need to agree how the agenda for the meeting is set, and what will happen if a discussion runs over time. In some cases, a supervisor may need to bring a discussion gently, but firmly, to a close. It is vital to finish sessions on time, allowing time at the end of the session to review what has happened and plan the actions to be taken prior to the next session.

Clinical supervision does not necessarily involve records; however, this can help in ensuring that the arrangements remain formal. It is perhaps wise for the supervisee to take responsibility for safe storage of these, and it should be stressed that these should not include patient/client details.

Clinical supervision dynamics

An organizational and departmental culture may have a direct impact on your success as a clinical supervisor (Grant, 2000). Problematic dynamics can occur when there is a perceived lack of collaboration or involvement on the part of the manager, supervisor or supervisee, three major stakeholders in any implementation of clinical supervision (Figure 4.3).

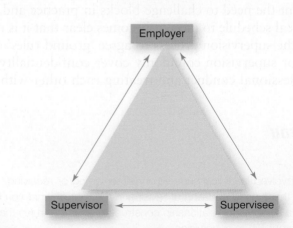

Figure 4.3   The three-cornered contract in clinical supervision, (adapted from English, 1975)

In the three-cornered contract illustrated above, the desired situation exists where the contract and expectations are clear on all sides, all role definitions are clear and there are no hidden agendas.

Problematic dynamics can include the following:

- Although supervisor and supervisee feel that they are on the same wavelength, both feel distant from their employers, who do not seem interested in supporting clinical supervision.

- Employer and supervisors are clear about their goals and actions, although there is considerable distance between them and the supervisee. The supervisee may be reluctant to take up the supervision opportunity and may view the supervisors as having a management-oriented evaluative role.

- The supervisor is seen as an outsider by both the employer and supervisee, leaving the supervisor feeling both psychologically isolated and that they value clinical supervision differently from others.

Despite these potential problems in implementing clinical supervision and other clinical facilitation roles, health care professions have shown increasing interest in receiving clinical supervision and reflecting upon the nature of their own learning needs.

Clinical supervisory discussions can cover a whole range of subject or topic areas, and this is likely to vary considerably between staff. There are, however, six broad areas that are often discussed:

- clinical working or a particular case – reflecting on work experiences and developing new skills
- management and organizational working – changes in work practices, managing time and workload, staff relationships
- confidence building – exploring past actions and affirming these
- professional development – career advice, locating learning experiences/opportunities
- educational support – discussing how to coach and work with others
- personal matters and interpersonal problems affecting clinical working.

We will explore how a questioning style can be adopted in the online bonus feature attached to this chapter.

Approaches to clinical supervision

There are different styles of clinical supervision, drawing on ideas from both leadership and teamwork. One widespread approach is to describe a continuum between a highly directive, proactive style (where the supervisor takes the decisions) and a more hands-off style (where the supervisee or group takes the decisions).

Reflective activity

Are you more comfortable in a situation where a supervisor is:

● directing and taking decisions
● co-ordinating and sharing the decisions with you
● space giving and letting you take the decisions?

It may be that, as the practitioner becomes more experienced, the style of the clinical supervisor should move along the range of the continuum from 'directing' towards 'space giving'. There is a range of skills and qualities that a clinical supervisor may require in order to achieve successful supervision.

Over to you

Assess yourself against each of the skills in Table 4.1. For each skill give yourself a score between 1 and 5, where 1 = a skill you need to develop and 5 = a skill you feel confident in.

Table 4.1 Skills and qualities of a clinical supervisor					
Skill/Quality	1	2	3	4	5
Facilitating reflection on practice					
Demonstrating effective non-verbal listening skills, e.g. eye-contact, prompts, body posture, managing the physical environment					
Demonstrating effective verbal listening skills, e.g. verbal prompts, open-ended questions, repeating key words, checking impressions					
Giving negative feedback					
Giving positive feedback					
Inspiring confidence in others					
Being emotionally supportive and restorative					
Dealing critically with personal and professional dilemmas					
Acting as a professional resource					
Self-disclosing appropriately					

(Continued)

Table 4.1 Skills and qualities of a clinical supervisor (*Continued*)					
Skill/Quality	**1**	**2**	**3**	**4**	**5**
Setting mutually agreed goals					
Preventing dependency in a professional relationship					
Dealing effectively with issues of unsafe/ unprofessional conduct					
Demonstrating a clear understanding of ethical rights and responsibilities					
Being self-critical					
Able to evaluate					

Adapted from East Somerset NHS Trust *Clinical Supervision: Theoretical and practical approaches to the supervision of clinical practice.* East Somerset NHS Trust, Yeovil, Somerset.

Within your review of your own skills, you may have identified dealing critically with professional dilemmas and challenging another's practice as areas for further development. Some practitioners may be less open to new ideas, and you may need to challenge someone about an aspect of their practice or in relation to the clinical supervision sessions themselves. For example, a supervisor may need to challenge the supervisee over:

- problems about how the supervisee is behaving towards a patient/client
- prejudice towards a particular client group
- problems about the way they are behaving with other health care colleagues
- errors of judgement in their professional practice
- failing to work to their professional code of conduct
- arriving late or failing to make a session altogether without an appropriate reason
- behaving inappropriately during a session
- behaving antagonistically towards another member of the supervision group.

In any of these cases, it is the responsibility of a clinical supervisor to act. In many cases, it can be enough to use the approaches to giving negative feedback, discussed earlier in this chapter. This may be sufficient for the supervisee to admit to the problem and to look to find a solution; in other cases, the supervisee may have a 'block' and change may not happen. If so, you may need to challenge the supervisee, and to confront their personal and professional blocks.

There are potential risks if we ignore the need to challenge another's practice. Hoping the issue/problem will go away and doing nothing can lead to the possibility that the situation will build up into a crisis. Challenging a colleague has the potential to be either a destructive or a productive force (see Table 4.2). If the situation is handled appropriately and sensitively, with the problem being aired openly, the supervisor and supervisee are enabled to listen to each other and to develop new solutions.

Table 4.2 Characteristics of productive and destructive challenges	
Productive challenges	**Destructive challenges**
Focus is on interests and facts instead of needs	Needs and personalities are emphasized
Lead to a long-term change	Lead to short-term solutions for longstanding problems
Are approached in an open manner	Are about face saving and the preservation of power
Help both supervisee and supervisor to reach their objectives	Supervisee and supervisor talk past one another, so that messages are not understood correctly and neither's objectives are reached
Are built on a bedrock of a good supervisory relationship	Damage the relationship and have the habit of being repeated

There are a number of approaches or ways to organize clinical supervision including:

- one-to-one expert supervision (own discipline)
- one-to-one expert supervision (different discipline)
- one-to-one peer supervision
- group supervision (facilitated by a supervisor)
- peer-group supervision (may or may not be facilitated by a supervisor)
- network supervision (a group of practitioners come together from a range of localities, e.g. senior nurses from Special Care Baby Units across a region)
- cascade supervision (usually based on management arrangements, e.g. Band 7 practitioners provide clinical supervision for the Band 6 practitioners and so on).

Over to you

Each of the above approaches to clinical supervision has advantages as well as possible problems. Take three of the approaches (choose the ones you see being used more commonly in your own area of practice) and, thinking about your own locality, write down the strengths and possible problems with these forms of supervision.

Strengths and potential problems of individual supervision

Individual supervision has a number of strengths but also potential problems (see Table 4.3). In clinical supervision, the 'helping professional' takes on a role of clinical supervisor and care needs to be taken that the relationship does not take the form of a client-practitioner. Discussions about client/patient working may lead to analysis of transference **and** countertransference. Transference is the experiencing of feelings, drives, attitudes and fantasies, and defences towards a person in the present which do not befit that person, but are a repetition of reactions originating in regard to significant persons (for example, mother, father, sibling) from early childhood, unconsciously displaced onto figures in the present. Understanding and responding to transference and countertransference is an important part of working relationships and can help in the identification of 'blind spots' for clinical supervisors and supervisees. These processes may also be paralleled in the supervisory relationship (Playle and Mullarkey, 1998). However, we would suggest that clinical supervisors think carefully and use these concepts cautiously if these interpretations are to be helpful in clinical supervision and goal attainment and, more importantly, ensure that this does not cause harm.

Transference
In the traditional psychoanalytical sense, transference is defined as feeling or acting towards somebody (e.g. a helping professional) in a way that relates more to another past or present relationship

Counter-transference
This occurs the other way, with the helping professional relating unconsciously to the client, based on past or current relationships

Table 4.3 Strengths and potential problems of individual supervision	
Strengths	**Possible Problems**
Time dedicated to one supervisee, so effective working can be speedily achieved	Can be difficult to address a breakdown in the relationship
Able to create clear and focused objectives for the supervisee	Supervisee and supervisor can more easily collude, and avoid challenging existing poor practice
Input from one direction (supervisor)	Can foster dependency in the supervisee
Personalized supervisory discussions	Less diverse range of ways of working/suggestions for the supervisee
Supervisee can work at own pace	The effectiveness of the supervisor – working is less open to evaluation
Supervisory session can be contained to around an hour and is easier to arrange as only two people involved	Transference issues may hamper clinical supervision, if unresolved
Less competitive environment	Can become a comfortable chat
Development in supervision can be easily monitored and is likely to be consistent	Evaluation and feedback is only one person's perspective

Strengths and potential problems of group supervision

Faugier and Butterworth (1992) suggest that one-to-one supervision tends to be the most frequently used approach; however, group supervision can be equally valuable (see Table 4.4). The choice of approach will depend upon a

Table 4.4 Strengths and potential problems of group supervision	
Strengths	**Possible Problems**
Emotionally supportive atmosphere from peers	Individual's needs may not be addressed – not all are suited to group work
Can encourage experimentation with care interventions	Group members may work at varying paces
Input from many directions, e.g. supervisor and other group members	Individuals may not have the time within a session to discuss their issue or can chose to 'hide' within the group
Some supervisory discussions not about individual supervisee needs	Supervisory session needs to be longer, around two hours – difficult to arrange as a group of people is involved
Learning achieved through listening, discussing others' work and reflecting on the problems they face can be valuable	The effectiveness of the supervisor – working is less open to evaluation
Cost effective in time of the supervisor and group members	Can become a competitive environment owing to group dynamics
Less likely for dependency towards the supervisor to occur	May be lack of time for group members with large caseloads
Evaluation and feedback given from a number of people	Can be used as a 'dumping ground', where issues outside of the individuals' controls are focused on
Risk taking can be higher in group setting	Can be pressure to conform, e.g. 'group think', and newcomers can find it difficult to join
Issues arising from within the group can be addressed	Lessening of confidentiality can be a problem
Reduces the power of supervisor	Individual development in supervision can be more difficult to monitor

number of factors, including personal choice, access to supervision, length of experience, qualifications, and the availability of supervisory groups. In the last 'Over to you' activity you probably identified that it is important that group supervision establishes effective group working, which can take longer to achieve than in a one-to-one situation. Group supervision requires facilitation skills and an appreciation of group dynamics: for instance, an understanding of the stages of group development – forming, storming, norming, performing and adjourning (Tuckman and Jensen, 1977) – see Figure 4.4.

It is essential that there is stability in the clinical supervisory relationships in order to develop mutual trust, respect and security: qualities that are

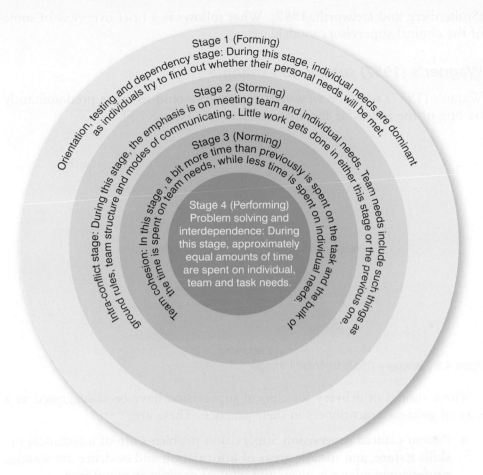

Figure 4.4   The stages of group development, (reflects the thinking of Tuckman and Jensen, 1977)

developed during long-term relationships. This can be difficult to achieve within the clinical supervision group, where turnover of membership can pose a threat to the functional dynamics of the group. Tuckman and Jensen (1977) added the final stage – adjourning – to signal that some groups do not survive long term. As members become aware of the group's demise, they may experience sadness and remorse, and sometimes find it difficult to disengage from task behaviours.

Models of clinical supervision

There are three main categories of models of clinical supervision (Faugier and Butterworth, 1992). First, there are those that describe supervision in relation to the main functions of the supervisory relationship and its constituents (Wagner, 1957; Heron, 1989); secondly, there are models that describe the main functions of the role (Proctor, 1987), and, thirdly, there are developmental models, which emphasize the process of the supervisory relationship

(Stoltenberg and Delworth, 1987). What follows is a brief overview of some of the clinical supervisory models.

Wagner's (1957) supervision triangle

Wagner (1957) took the view that supervisors tend to focus predominantly on one of the following three parameters (see Figure 4.5).

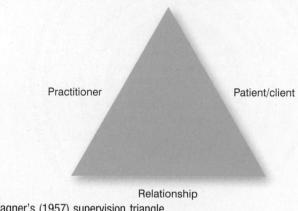

Figure 4.5   Wagner's (1957) supervision triangle

Three modes of delivery for clinical supervision have been suggested as a way of guiding practitioners in their practice. These are:

- **Patient-centred supervision** Supervision problems are of a technical or skills nature, and specific areas of information and evidence are sought, professional advice is given and clinical practice is monitored.
- **Clinical-centred supervision** The focus is on unseen, unheard or unspoken components of practice through reflection on clinical events. The practitioner is encouraged to look at the dynamics involved and the factors influencing their clinical practice.
- **Process-centred supervision** This concentrates on the processes of events between a patient, family members, colleagues, and a practitioner and their supervisor. Analogies are made between interactions that take place with the supervisor, and interactions between the patient and supervisee, sometimes termed mirroring or paralleling. This demands specific high-level supervisor skills.

Obviously, focusing on one of these at the expense of the others could limit the usefulness of the supervisory interactions.

Heron's (1989) six category intervention analysis

John Heron (1989) proposed a taxonomy for the analysis and categorization of interventions employed during counselling, which has been used as a way to review clinical supervision interventions. The six main forms of intervention are of two types: authoritative and facilitative.

Forms of intervention (Heron, 1989)

Authoritative

- **Prescriptive** – the supervisor directs the supervisee by giving advice and direction.
- **Informative** – the supervisor provides information and instructs the supervisee.
- **Confrontative** – the supervisor challenges the beliefs or behaviour of the supervisee. Such confrontation does not imply aggression, rather it invites the supervisee to consider some aspect of their work or themselves that they have previously taken for granted.

Facilitative

- **Cathartic** – the supervisor attempts to help the supervisee move on through the expression of thoughts or emotions previously unacknowledged or expressed.
- **Catalytic** – the supervisor focuses on helping the supervisee become increasingly self-directive and reflective. They aim to 'bump up' the developmental and professional level of the supervisee.
- **Supportive** – the supervisor attempts to reinforce the confidence of the supervisee through focusing on their areas of competence, and attending to what they did well.

Sloan and Watson (2001) suggest that all of the intervention categories should be utilized within clinical supervision to realize the potential potency of Heron's framework.

Over to you

Seek the agreement of all parties involved in your supervision to record a clinical supervision interaction (make sure that this is kept confidential) then review this, filling in the following clinical supervision recording chart (Table 4.5) to show every time that the supervisor communicates. Mark which category the intervention falls within. Then discuss the review findings with all participants in the clinical supervision when you next meet.

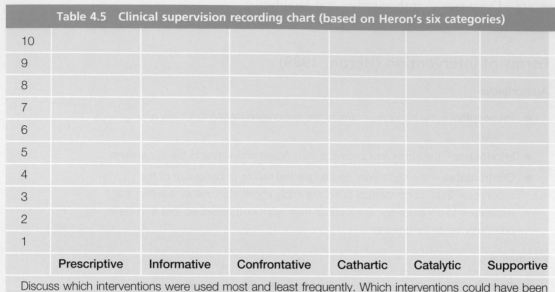

	Prescriptive	Informative	Confrontative	Cathartic	Catalytic	Supportive
10						
9						
8						
7						
6						
5						
4						
3						
2						
1						

Table 4.5   Clinical supervision recording chart (based on Heron's six categories)

Discuss which interventions were used most and least frequently. Which interventions could have been used more to get the most from the clinical supervision episode?

Proctor's (1987) three function interactive model

Kadushin (1992) looked at supervision in social work and identified three main functions of supervision: administrative, educational and supportive. This way of thinking about supervision has become generally accepted, and Proctor (1987) adapted the model. The administrative function was changed to a professional or 'normative' function that includes the provision of quality control. The educative or 'formative' function was enlarged; this function enables the development of skills, understanding and abilities by reflecting on and exploring the person's work experience. The supportive or 'restorative' function provides support to enable the person to deal with what has happened and to move on.

A way of remembering this clinical supervisory model is to think of ESP.

- Educational – to further develop knowledge and skills
- Supportive – to ensure that practitioner stability and boundaries are effective
- Professional – to maintain safe practice and satisfactory standards of care.

This framework helps in directing the balance of interactions within a clinical supervisory meeting and is also useful in evaluating the effectiveness of the relationship. However, the way that these functions are depicted tends to suggest that supervisees are in deficit, with it being the job of the clinical supervisor to help them to put things right. If this is the way that clinical supervision is viewed, the supervisor can easily slip into acting on, or upon behalf of, their supervisee.

Hawkins and Shohet (1989) have identified the primary aspects of supervision as:

- to provide a regular space for the supervisees to reflect upon the content and process of their work (Educational)
- to develop understanding and skills within the work setting (Educational)
- to receive information and another perspective concerning one's work (Educational, Supportive)
- to receive both content and process feedback (Educational, Supportive)
- to be validated and supported both as a person and as a practitioner (Supportive)
- to ensure that as a person and as a practitioner one is not left to carry unnecessarily difficult problems and projects alone (Supportive)
- to have space to explore and express personal distress, re-stimulation, transference or countertransference that may be brought up by the work (Administrative/Professional)
- to plan and utilize their personal and professional resources better (Administrative/Professional)
- to be pro-active rather than re-active (Administrative/Professional)
- to ensure quality of work (Administrative/Professional, Supportive).

Stoltenberg and Delworth's (1987) integrative development model

This model focuses on the content and process of supervision that change as the supervisee progresses in their practice:

- Stage 1 – There is reliance on the supervisor, and much of the content of supervision is based on role modelling and influencing.
- Stage 2 – This is an exploratory phase when the supervisee starts to take risks in the development of their practice and the supervisor challenges blocks and blindspots.
- Stage 3 – The supervisee takes up a position of autonomy, working on their skills and knowledge acquisition independently, and looks to the supervisor to enlarge their understanding of broader professional issues.

Although this model shows three stages that appear to progress from one to another, a practitioner might be at Stage 3 for much of their practice but also at Stage 1 for a new clinical case that they have not dealt with before.

Even though clinical supervision models vary considerably in their approach to clinical supervision, they have in common themes like supervisor– supervisee–client interaction, support, educational development, equality, shared responsibility, and the importance of a good interpersonal relationship.

Using solution-focused techniques in clinical supervision

Solution-focused clinical supervision offers a simple structure for the supervisory relationship. Solution-focused clinical supervision makes the assumption that the supervisee has the answers within her or himself and by focusing on their effective patterns of behaviour the answers will be uncovered (Fowler *et al.*, 2007). Incorporating solution-focused techniques into clinical supervision enhances the supervisor's range of options with which to help the supervisees to determine positive actions rather than dwelling on problems. Waskett (2006) has identified 'spacious simplicity', a term that comes from a basic attitude of mutual respect; combined with the intention of moving forward. There are a number of techniques used within solution-based therapies that are applicable in the supervisory relationship, including:

- The use of scales
- Focused questions
- Looking for exceptions and assumptions
- Constructive feedback
- Follow-up tasks (George *et al.*, 1999).

This framework of methods assist the clinical supervisor to engage collaboratively with supervisee, encouraging reflection on practice and a focus on solutions. Solution-focused clinical supervision is underpinned by both humanistic and behavioural models, in that it values the supervisor-supervisee relationship as the basis for growth, whilst helping the supervisee to plan and take steps forward. Solution-focused therapy was developed in the 1980s, by de Shazer (1985) as an option falling within the umbrella of 'talking therapies'. The approach is brief and works on solutions with a minimal emphasis on problems. Attention is devoted to developing the person's preferred future or goal and what will need to happen and be available to achieve this. This approach to therapy is also useful within clinical supervisory contexts.

Fowler *et al.* (2007) suggest the following example questions as a framework for clinical supervision, suggesting the role of the clinical supervisor as 'curious inquirer':

- So what did it take to do that?
- What helped you to achieve that?
- How did you do that?
- How did you get through that time/experience/deal with that difficulty?
- What did you learn about yourself managing to do that?
- What do you think that might have taught others about you?

There are a number of techniques that can help the supervisee focus on the positive e.g. using a 0-10 scale, where 10 represents absolute best achievement of the supervisee's goals and zero is the worst-case scenario. The supervisee uses the scale to assess their current position and satisfaction with this, and identifies their preferred position. Use of a 'miracle question' can determine preferred futures or goals. When discussing preferred futures with students, it is enormously helpful to make use of the 'miracle question'. This is probably the central and key strategy to the solution-focused approach. It is a creative way of eliciting the description of a preferred future and the question can be phrased as follows: imagine that when you are asleep tonight a miracle happens – it is almost as if a magic wand is waved over you and the problem or difficulty you are currently experiencing is eliminated. You are not aware of what has happened when you wake up, but you notice the changes. What is it that you notice when you wake up, and as you continue through your day, that lets you know that this miracle has occurred? The student is then encouraged to be very specific about describing all the changes in detail, elaborating further on their preferred future. The supervisee is asked to consider if there are times when aspects of the miracle are already happening (exceptions). At the start of each clinical supervision session the supervisee is asked 'What is better?' as opposed to 'How are things?', and at the end of session provides a summary of the supervisee's strengths, skills and resources.

MANAGING THE REALITIES IN PRACTICE

As with other relationships which occur in the workplace, trying to engage with a preceptor and managing competing demands can be challenging. Consideration needs to be given when planning how to meet and discuss experience and practice. Individuals may be in the same unit but not perhaps in the same team therefore agreeing early on how to proceed and link up will ensure that expectations are clear. As previously stated there are similarities within the role of mentor, preceptor and clinical supervisor. It is interesting to note that Mooney (2007b) discovered that practitioners during the initial stages of qualification, recognized that as pre-registration students they had unmet needs and were isolated at times. She recommends attention to these in order to benefit them post-registration.

Over to you

Read this article:
   Hughes, A.J. and Fraser, D.M. (2011) Sink or Swim: The experience of newly qualified midwives in England. *Midwifery,* **27**(3): 382–386.
   Reflect on your experience as a newly registered practitioner or preceptor. Did you have any similar thoughts?

Clinical supervision is equally demanding for both supervisors and supervisees, bringing to those involved additional obligations and responsibilities if a strong supervisory relationship is to be established and maintained. The early phases of the clinical supervision relationship make a significant contribution

The supervisory relationship

- Generosity – in time, and being prepared to give, both emotionally and intellectually
- Rewarding – offering praise and encouragement
- Openness – to feelings, as well as providing practical skills development
- Willingness to learn – from each other
- Thoughtful and thought provoking
- Humanity – treating those involved as individuals with whom it is a privilege to work
- Sensitivity – awareness of problems
- Uncompromising – bringing rigour to the process, encouraging high standards of work
- Orientation – recognizing when viewpoints may conflict and when professional opinions may conflict with the needs of the patient/client
- Trust – those involved need to maintain safety

to the overall efficacy of clinical supervision (Sloan, 2005). The development of the relationship from the perspective of the supervisee will have an impact on issues they wish to disclose, confidence in the process has to be earned.

The supervisee and supervisor need to be able to communicate their feelings and thoughts clearly and honestly. There has to be a willingness to listen to the other person's point of view and to take on board their thoughts and feelings. It can be helpful to allow some time after the discussion for the supervisee to accept the challenge to their practice, so that they can separate their emotions and initial feelings about the challenge from the practical aspects of the problem. If a supervisee reacts in a manner that you were not expecting, it helps to realize that we cannot always know what 'buttons' are being pressed in the other person.

You may find the following useful when challenging another's practice:

- Remember that by demonstrating a willingness to confront difficult issues in another's practice we are doing so to encourage resolution of the problem.

- Listen to the other person carefully, to their words and observe their non-verbal signals, without interruption. This shows that you value the other person's viewpoint.

- Repeat and/or summarize the other person's discussion as this demonstrates the attention you have paid, shows active listening and may allow anything that you have misunderstood to be corrected.

- Reflect back the feelings of the other person, which may show them that you care about the feelings aroused: for example, 'It sounds like you're feeling annoyed'.

- Work with the supervisee to tackle or resolve the problem, avoiding interrupting or jumping in to judge or dismiss their ideas. (Writing notes at this point may help both of you.)
- Be aware of your communication style; tone of voice (try to speak calmly and evenly), use positive body language (give eye contact, nod, and do not fold your arms); don't interrupt but allow space for exploration of the issue, and ask open questions to encourage information to surface.

TOP TIPS

- Establish a safe physical, social and psychological environment
- Focus on sustaining and developing practice
- Explore and clarify thinking
- Share information, experience and skills
- Confront personal and professional blocks
- Encourage the involvement and, where appropriate, empowerment of patients, clients and relatives
- Maintain high standards of practice
- Give clear feedback
- Explore professional accountability
- Facilitate understanding of team and organizational contracts

In this chapter we have explored two different methods of professional support, how these can be approached and the benefits of engaging in them.

RAPID RECAP

Check your progress so far by working through each of the following questions.

1 What are the main differences between mentorship and preceptorship?

2 What issues need to be decided in order to formalize a preceptorship programme?

3 Define 'clinical supervision' and name two models/frameworks for clinical supervision.

4 Why are ground rules necessary within clinical supervision?

If you have difficulty with any of these questions, read through the section again to refresh your understanding before moving on.

CHAPTER 5
IDENTIFYING INDIVIDUAL LEARNING NEEDS

LEARNING OBJECTIVES

By the end of this chapter you should be able to:

● explain the factors that affect your learning

● undertake an assessment of your learning style

● appreciate the need to balance individual learning needs with job/role requirements

● discuss the structure and process of developing a learning contract.

Bonus features for this chapter available on the book's website

INTRODUCTION

In this chapter, we focus on individual learning. Each learner should be viewed as an individual; plans and opportunities tailored to their individual needs even when they may be two people at the same stage in the same environment. A key component of supporting practice learning is being able to identify learning outcomes to provide a rich yet pertinent learning experience. You will think about individual learning stories and the factors that affect these, such as learning styles and motivation. We will also look at how individual learning needs (knowledge and skills) can be identified, objectives set and a plan carried out. As many students and qualified health care practitioners work within the NHS, we have included a brief overview of the Knowledge and Skills Framework, which is now used throughout the NHS, and shown how this can be integrated into an individual learning contract.

INDIVIDUAL LEARNING STORIES

The best way to start thinking about the individual learner's needs is to consider past learning experiences. When we meet someone for the first time, we often exchange information about where we work and about our family and friends so that we learn something about each other, even though this is usually on quite a superficial level and only gives a small insight into the person. Examining personal learning stories can be a much more illuminating process. When a learner feels comfortable talking about their story, they can illuminate important points about learning preferences and 'blindspots'. This is useful for the mentor as both the learner and their mentor can take into account the different learning histories that participants bring with them.

Reflective activity

Draw a line on a blank sheet of paper, starting with you at age five and continuing to the present day. At various points on this line, identify where you felt your learning experience was significant. For instance, this may be when you first started your health care professional qualification. When you place a point on the line, jot down why there was a 'ramping up' of learning at that time. Then reflect on what this has told you about your 'learning story'.

Health care careers are often explained through mileposts that include a mix of job changes and personal family events. The sense of career capital created by professional qualifications, a career structure and occupational identity means that health care professionals often return to work following a break for personal, such as family, reasons. When people talk about the influences on their lives, they often use the metaphor of a journey in which certain key decisions and experiences determine its route thereafter. Many career decisions are felt to be opportunistic and affected by chance (Wigens, 2004). Looking back on the last reflective activity, you may have felt that it helped to 'flesh out' your learning journey.

Decisions affecting whether you start your health care course, or perhaps choose not to commence a course at another time, are likely to be linked to your home or personal circumstances (Smith and Topping, 2001; Wigens, 2004). Bowden (2008) found that personal issues were one of the reasons cited by students who had considered leaving their course, this largely resulted from their course impacting on their time or upsetting their emotional equlilibrium.

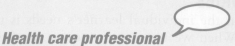

Health care professional

Physiotherapist – emergency admission department

Where I worked before, courses were unheard of. Managers didn't push you to do any non-essential course. But here, more recently, courses have become much more available. It's very good; there's so much out there. I've done the leadership module, and started on my Master's degree; I did the change management module and the research methods. Then I became pregnant and I haven't picked it up again yet. My family life is very important: I don't want to leave my little girl. The courses made me think about how I do things, especially when I was doing the leadership one.

Working in an area that makes it possible to access post-registration courses increases individual learning opportunities. Success in pre- and post-registration studies appear to be linked to the motivation and hard work of the student, their personal life situation, and the support given by the employer in terms of funding or study leave. Nurses talk about critical incidents or informal social/group interactions within their career that act as catalysts to their professional learning (Wigens, 2004). Individual motivators to learn, knowledge of oneself as a learner, and a disposition to learn, as well as service area benefits, are seen as the key to successful continuous professional development (CPD), and successful personal development plans are negotiated with all these elements in mind.

The following case study account is from a staff nurse working in an Accident and Emergency Department; it identifies many of the factors that are linked to lifelong learning in nursing. Read the account and identify key factors that affected this staff nurse's individual lifelong learning.

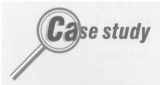

Case study

Factors affecting lifelong learning

I was just plodding along, getting sluggish and fed up with nursing. The conversion to a registered nurse course helped because as an enrolled nurse I couldn't go any further. I know I was very close to leaving nursing if I hadn't got on the conversion course. I'm a lot happier now I can do more things, like plastering, and I wouldn't have been able to do an A & E course as an enrolled nurse. The modules I've been doing on the A & E course make me see how little I know about certain things. I know a little bit about most things and I use the profiles to increase my knowledge.

The course has highlighted what I want to go on and find out a bit more about. Things that go on in the department mean that I want to learn more about certain things. The conversion course wasn't what I was expecting; I was hoping to learn more anatomy and physiology. But then I've gone out and done it myself. I see myself as staying in A & E and

I'd like to do my Registered Mental Nurse training to use in the department. It's not just the work here that has led to an interest in mental health, but I've had involvement with people close to me with mental health problems in my personal life. I'm also told that I'm very good with the suicide patients. I find time to talk to them, and a lot of the time that's all they want. In my personal life I've had a lot of things to cope with from a very young age and that's made me, I think, a very strong person anyway.

From reading the previous account of the factors affecting an individual's lifelong learning, you will have identified a complex range of interrelated aspects. You probably also noted this in your reflection on your own lifelong learning. Self-development, although appearing individual, is also social in nature.

INDIVIDUAL CONTINUOUS PROFESSIONAL DEVELOPMENT

There is a long history of researchers studying the CPD activities of professionals: Ryan (2003), Banning and Stafford (2008) and Schostak *et al.* (2010). Banning and Stafford (2008) found that community practitioners viewed CPD positively, with development needs being identified through reflection. The need for CPD has been heightened by the realization that a professional's claim to possess specific, advanced knowledge can only be made in the light of evidence that professional education is ongoing and effective. Organizational and managerial reforms demand that practitioners be self-motivated regarding their personal and professional development.

Illeris (2007) presents a model of learning triangulated around two axis: one concerned with content and incentive - the 'what' is learnt and 'motivation for learning it' respectively; and the other concerned with interaction between the individual and the environment (see Figure 5.1 on the next page). Illeris suggests that the learner's knowledge and abilities are developed through the content dimension, the mental energy or motivation required to achieve this from the incentive element; both being activated by impulses from the interactive processes. Central to the incentive dimension is that the learning related challenges should be in relative balance with the learner's interests and qualifications. He feels that learning is always underpinned by the context: the social and societal influences. Students in and on interprofessional health care courses can have very broadly harmonizing aims: to be able to practice as a competent practitioner and to increase their knowledge and understanding.

Within one case site, the outcome of engaging in CPD was assessed in terms of both the visible changes in an individual's nursing practice and CPD's ability to develop careers by preparing nurses for promotion (Wigens, 2004). It can be difficult to determine the full impact of individual CPD

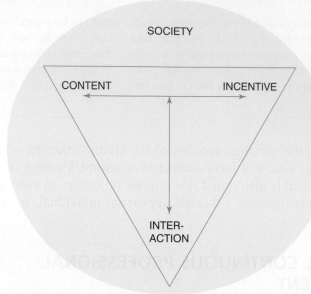

Figure 5.1   Illeris' Three dimensions of learning, (adapted from Illeris, 2007, p. 26)

activities on health care practice as the development of the individual is inextricably linked with their own personal development and clinical/professional development. Individual motivations are explored in the next section.

MOTIVATION

The concept of motivation seems to provide an answer to the question, 'What makes us do the things we do?' Motivation is what leads us to behave, act or learn in specific, purposeful ways. One of the pioneers of motivation research, Houle (1961), identified three categories of adult learner:

- goal-oriented (pursuing identified objectives)
- learning-oriented (learning for the love of it)
- activity-oriented (learning for reasons unconnected with objectives but task related).

These categories are still largely accepted although it is now common to reduce them to a simple dichotomy – learning for instrumental motives (to achieve specific goals) or for intrinsic motives (learning for its own sake). However, this instrumental-versus-intrinsic division is perhaps too simplistic as people often have mixed motives for learning. One could focus on individual characteristics, such as learning styles and motivation, or on 'attractors' and 'deterrents' affecting participation in continuing education activities, assessing the role that workplace challenges and opportunities play in individuals' learning activities.

Maslow (1954) defined a hierarchy of needs that should be satisfied before effective learning can occur (Figure 5.2). He suggested that these needs must be attended to in their hierarchical order. They are:

- physiological – to be fed and watered
- safety – freedom from excessive anxiety
- social – the need to be loved and cared for, respected as a person
- self-esteem – skills mastered; recognition by others
- self-fulfilment – personal achievement, freedom to take responsibility, be creative and develop.

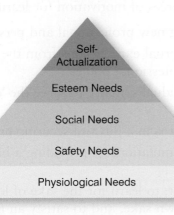

Figure 5.2 Maslow's hierarchy of needs, (adapted from Maslow, 2012)

Reflective activity

Look at the following quote from an on-call radiographer, working a weekend duty.

"The staff member who was on a 9-5 had been in theatre all day leaving me to work single-handed. I then had to call the standby radiographer in who lived 45 minutes away and they got held up in traffic. While I was trying to catch up, I got called for an urgent mobile X-ray on one of the wards. It was a very long day and I knew I wasn't stopping to drink or eat. I had to make a conscious effort because I nearly passed out on the unit and it was just because I was so tired, I wasn't drinking. I hadn't had anything to eat and I was totally exhausted. Sometimes you really have to make yourself sit down."

Do you think this radiographer's comments have any connection to Maslow's hierarchy of need and its link with motivations to learn? Do any of the factors identified by Maslow affect your motivation to learn in clinical settings? What needs do you think need to be met before clinical learning is likely to occur?

When health care practitioners perceive a need to learn something, they are generally capable of working very hard, but as adults with many roles (e.g. spouse, parent, employee, student) they are often time-conscious learners. Therefore, most want to meet their educational goals as directly, quickly, and efficiently as possible. The challenge is to create a non-threatening atmosphere in which practitioners have permission to learn and are expected to share in the responsibility for their learning. Establishing 'adult-to-adult' rapport and using positive non-verbal and verbal communication can help to create the right atmosphere. The mentor needs to deal with the whole person, addressing the learner as an equal and employing an informally structured approach. Adult learners appreciate supervisors who share appropriate information and are approachable and accessible.

Factors that act as sources of motivation for learning include:

- meeting and making new professional and personal relationships
- complying with external expectations from the higher education institute and the professional bodies
- improving the individual's ability to serve the 'community of practice' or clinical team
- achieving higher status in a job and securing professional advancement
- an escape, or for stimulation, by providing a break in the routine of home or work
- for cognitive interest: to learn for the sake of learning, seeking knowledge for its own sake, and to satisfy an inquiring mind.

How that energy is directed and at what level may be a direct result of the social context of each individual learner. When the presence of a group motivates an individual to pursue a particular behaviour, it is called social facilitation. If the nature of the task or discussion within the group is interesting, interactive and involving, it is more likely to motivate the individual to achieve. This is especially true if the individual feels a personal affinity or particular talent for the task.

Reflective activity

Think about your recent areas of interest and about learning situations where you put in more effort than you needed to. What was it about that particular area of practice learning that motivated you?

We can easily get into 'habits' regarding our learning; habitual action refers to what has been previously learnt and becomes automatic through frequent use. A habit is at the intersection between knowledge, skill and desire (Covey, 2004a) and is non-reflective:

- Knowledge is 'what to do and why'.
- Skill is 'how to do'.
- Desire is 'motivation and the want to do'.

Knowledge, skill and desire have to interrelate for effective habits to develop. For example, you may have noted that you are a poor listener regarding peer worker problems. You may know that you need to listen and you may know how to listen, but if you don't have the desire to listen it won't be a habit in your life.

Seven main habits of highly effective people (Covey, 2004a)

Habit 1 – Be Proactive
Habit 2 – Begin with the end in mind
Habit 3 – Put first things first
Habit 4 – Think win/win
Habit 5 – Seek first to understand then to be understood
Habit 6 – Synergize
Habit 7 – Sharpen the saw

According to Covey (2004a), habits 1, 2 and 3 deal with self-mastery, that is, moving from dependence (you do it) to independence (I do it). These habits are seen as 'private victories', the essence of personal learning and growth: learning to define oneself, rather than relying purely on other people's opinions or by comparison to others. Private victories are viewed as the precursor to public victories. Habits 4, 5 and 6, are personality-oriented 'public victories', involving interdependence (we do it), teamwork, co-operation and communication. These habits foster improved relationships and the desire to rebuild important relationships. Habit 7 is one of renewal, and Covey (2004a) suggests that this should encircle all the other habits. A habit of continuous improvement and self-renewal is viewed as creating the upward spiral for growth. Reflecting on, and having an awareness of habits which reduce our ability to learn and that reduce our personal effectiveness, is required.

Since these habits were originally published Covey (2004b), has introduced an eighth habit, he says as a result of the challenges and changes we face in our personal and professional lives. The seven habits are still highly relevant, the greater the challenge the more relevant they become. However simply being 'effective' is now a given expectation, the new era demands greatness (Covey, 2004b). The 8th habit is – Find your voice and inspire others to find theirs. He says that this is the voice of human spirit; we think that this is particularly apt in today's health care environment and for us it reflects the shared responsibility that we have to display effective leadership behaviours.

The length of time that learner motivation can be sustained is variable, hence the usefulness of periodic reviews of progress through, for example, learning contracts or personal development plan review meetings. These not only help the learner to gain understanding of their achievements but also determine what action both the learner and the mentor/supervisor need to take.

LEARNING STYLES

Students may become more motivated to learn by knowing more about their own strengths and weaknesses as learners. The issue of learning styles has been partly addressed by the development of learning style models, of which there are many. Coffield *et al.* (2004) looked at 71 models of learning styles and then categorized 13 of these as major models. Within this chapter we have chosen to look at four of these, the last three of which are most commonly used within health care practice.

The four models presented briefly here take varying forms, being based on genetics (Dunn, 2003), personality type (Myers and McCaulley, 1998) and flexible learning preferences (Honey and Mumford, 1992; Kolb, 1984a). Some theorists have strong beliefs about the influence of genetics on fixed, inherited traits and about the interaction of personality and cognition. However, Dunn and Dunn's model (Dunn, 2003) does also acknowledge external factors, such as the immediate environment. Genetics-based models are rooted in ideas that styles should be worked with rather than changed. Other models of learning style are based on the relationship between self and experience with some paying greater attention to personal factors such as motivation, and others stressing the importance of environmental factors such as whether learning is collective or individual.

The Dunn and Dunn model

According to this model, a learning style is divided into five main elements that significantly influence what individuals learn; these are called stimuli. The stimulus elements are:

- environmental
- emotional
- sociological
- psychological
- physiological (Dunn, 2003, p. 2).

From these elements certain factors are thought to affect students' preferences (see Table 5.1, adapted from Coffield *et al.*, 2004).

Table 5.1 Factors affecting learning			
Element	**Factors**		
Environmental	Sound	Temperature	Light	Clinical area layout
Psychological	Likes to learn alone	Likes to learn in pairs	Likes to learn in a group	Likes to learn as part of a team
Emotional	Motivation	Need for structure	Degree of responsibility	Persistence
Physiological	Modality preference for VAKT[1] <ul><li>Visual</li><li>Auditory</li><li>Kinaesthetic/ Tactile</li></ul>	Physical functioning, e.g. intake of food and drink	Time of day	Mobility
Sociological	Learning group	Help and support from authority figures, e.g. mentor/ supervisor	Working alone or with peers	Motivation of the educator

[1]VAKT modalities are explained in the next section of this chapter.

The Dunn and Dunn model places a strong emphasis on biological and developmentally imposed characteristics. Each person's unique combination of preferences comprises their learning style. People who have no high or low preferences do not need 'matching' and can therefore adapt more easily to different learning activities. The model measures preferences rather than strengths and takes the view that we should not stigmatize different types of preference.

VAKT modalities

For effective learning to occur, a learner needs to feel comfortable with the methods used. Individuals can develop a preference for sending and receiving information through one sense over another. People more commonly prefer auditory or visual input; however, some people have a preference for kinaesthetic/tactile learning: learning that involves movement or touch. A preference for one type of learning over another can be identified:

- Visual learners prefer or enjoy graphic illustrations such as bar graphs to explain data; colour coding to highlight salient information; flowcharts within clinical guidelines; written material; wall charts that display points to be remembered; written outlines; drawings or designs to illustrate overhead presentations; looking at gestures or visuals.

- Auditory learners prefer or enjoy verbal presentation of new information; group discussions; fast-paced verbal exchanges of ideas; a good joke or story; verbal cues or mnemonic devices to help them remember information (e.g. ABC for Airway, Breathing, Circulation); oral reports of working.

- Kinesthetic/ tactile learners prefer or enjoy movement such as hands-on experience to learn a task; gesturing whilst making a point; role-play exercises; shaking hands when meeting or greeting people; trying new things without a lengthy explanation of the activity; frequent breaks; 'just doing it' rather than talking about it.

While it is thought that people have developed a preference for or have greater skill in processing one type of input over others, for most people information is processed simultaneously through multiple senses. In fact, the retention of learnt material is enhanced if the learner is able to use all senses.

Over to you

Identify your preferred learning modality. There are a number of tests available on line that you could try: for example, go to **www.businessballs.com** and select the learning styles VAK test.

The Myers-Briggs Type Indicator

The Myers-Briggs Type Indicator (MBTI) was developed in the early 1940s with the aim of making Jung's theory of human personality understandable and useful in everyday life (Myers and McCaulley, 1998). The MBTI looks at the descriptions of normally observed types based on personality factors.
The four bipolar scales of the MBTI are:

Extraversion (E)	Introversion (I)
Sensing (S)	Intuition (N)
Thinking (T)	Feeling (F)
Judging (J)	Perceiving (P)

From these eight personality features were developed 16 MBTI personality types: for example, ENTP (Extraversion, Intuition, Thinking, Perceiving).

Over to you

There are a range of online tools adapted from the MBTI that you could try. You can read more about Myers-Briggs personality types by looking at the section titled 'Myers-Briggs personality theory and MBTI types indicator' at **www.businessballs.com**.
    Do you agree with the findings, and what the type identified for you says?

Kolb's Learning Styles Inventory

The Learning Styles Inventory (LSI) was developed by David Kolb in the early 1970s and linked his theory of experiential learning to an instrument devised both to test his theory and to capture individual learning differences (Kolb, 1984a). He observed that some students had definite preferences for some activities: for example, some liked exercises but others preferred lectures (Figure 5.3). For Kolb (1984a), a learning style is not a fixed trait but a differential preference for learning, which changes slightly from situation to situation. However, he acknowledges that there is some longer-term stability in learning style. Kolb's four dominant learning styles are each located in a different quadrant of the cycle of experiential learning.

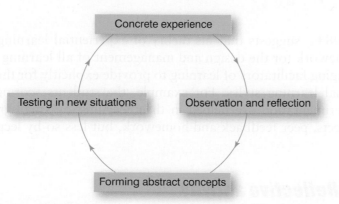

Figure 5.3   Diagram of Kolb's experiential learning cycle, (reflects the thinking of Kurt Lewin, 1942)

The learning cycle stages are:

1 concrete experience – feeling – having the experience
2 reflective observation – watching – reviewing the experience
3 abstract conceptualization – thinking – concluding from the experience
4 active experimentation – doing – planning the next stage

The four learning styles within Kolb's LSI are:

- **diverging** (concrete experience and reflective observation) – imaginative, interested in people, breadth of interests
- **assimilating** (abstract conceptualization and reflective observation) – theory creator, uses reasoning, able to handle abstract concepts
- **converging** (abstract conceptualization and active experimentation) – application to practice, depth of interest
- **accommodating** (concrete experience and active experimentation) – does things and takes risks, uses intuition to solve problems.

Kolb claimed that an appreciation of differing learning styles helps people to work more effectively in teams, resolve conflict, communicate at work and at home, and choose careers.

Over to you

Take a look at Chapter 2, pages 10–15 in Pearce, R. (2003) Foundations in Nursing and Health Care. *Profiles and Portfolios of Evidence*. Nelson Thornes, Cheltenham.

Identify your learning style using Kolb's LSI and think about how useful this could be to your learning in the future.

Kolb (1984a) suggests that his theory of experiential learning provides a useful framework for the design and management of all learning experiences by encouraging facilitators of learning to provide explicitly for the differences in individual learning styles. For example, the students scoring highest in active experimentation are helped in their learning by small-group discussions, projects, peer feedback and homework, but less so by lectures.

Reflective activity

Think about what learning approaches might be more successful within a clinical setting for each of the four learning style 'types'. Do you foresee any difficulties in a mentor/supervisor adapting a learning contract to 'fit' with the individual learning preferences?

Honey and Mumford's (1992) Learning Styles

Honey and Mumford (1992) acknowledged their intellectual debt to Kolb's (1984a) theory, but decided to produce their own learning style questionnaire and to change the unwieldy terms. They changed:

- diverger to reflector
- assimilator to theorist
- converger to pragmatist
- accommodator to activist.

Activists are said to have a preference for experiencing something immediately. They don't read the instruction manual first, but get straight on with the job. They want to do as many new things as possible and like short-term goals, often offering to lead. Reflectors prefer to 'wait and see', reviewing experiences or mulling over data. They take time to think before answering a question and can seem uncertain. Theorists like to build systems and to get first principles agreed. They speak in general rather than in concrete terms and draw conclusions in an objective manner. Pragmatists tend to be confident and energetic, taking short cuts and devising new ways of working. They enjoy problem solving and planning the next steps.

As all of these approaches to learning are viewed as useful, it is advocated that learners become proficient in all four. The complete learner would possess the ability to adopt all with equal facility, but there are not many such learners around, and most people have a preferred or dominant learning style, which can be explored by questionnaire (Honey and Mumford, 1992). Rather than ask people directly how they learn, Honey and Mumford designed a questionnaire, which probes general behavioural tendencies rather than learning.

Memletics

The memletics accelerated learning styles system recognizes that each person prefers different styles of learning (Memletics, 2004). These can be grouped into common ways: people often have a mix of styles but this can vary from a dominant style to different styles in different situations. There is no particular correct way, and you can develop ability in less dominant styles and further ability in more developed ones.

The styles are visual, aural, verbal, physical, logical, social and solitary (Memletics, 2004).

> ### Over to you
>
> You can carry out the test and plot your own learning styles graph online at http://www.learning-styles-online.com

Are the models useful?

Having looked at some of the learning style models and your own learning style, you are probably starting to form an opinion regarding the usefulness to you of this area of educational research. Learning styles have, for some, become an unquestioned part of their professional thinking and practice, allowing a quick and simple way of differentiating students, and this is understandable as the learning style literature promises practitioners a simple solution to the complex problems of improving the attainment, motivation and attitudes of individual students. Others consider these instruments to be unreliable and invalid and potentially damaging, as they may stereotype or label learners, so do not use them in their practice. We believe there is some merit in understanding an individual's learning preferences, but feel that this needs to be integrated into a holistic view of learning through practice.

INDIVIDUAL NEEDS ANALYSIS

Adult education views of learning tend to be built on a particular view of 'the self', which we touched upon in Chapter 2 when discussing andragogy. The idea of the adult learner as an autonomous self has become beyond question and the emphasis on learning within professional programmes is often about personal and professional change. Self-directed learning involves learners in finding out on their own initiative what they need to know. Such an active role is more likely to be adopted if the work is appropriately chosen and the learner is encouraged in their learning.

Identifying learning deficits can be difficult, because as health care deliverers we often seek to justify our actions rather than recognize errors or omissions. Everyone who works makes errors and omissions and the ability to acknowledge and work on these should be celebrated. The mentor needs to work with the learner's self-assessment and patient feedback to recognize and act on the areas requiring improvement.

CLINICAL CASE LOAD

Try using this example of a tool for identifying your learning needs. This activity should be carried out over the course of one shift or working day within clinical practice. Keep a notebook in your pocket and note any unmet patient needs that you recognize – the needs may be unmet because you did not have sufficient skills to deliver this aspect of care or treatment, or you may feel that you could have delivered care in a better way. This activity will enable you to identify an area that would benefit from further learning or development. Areas for learning should be grouped into:

- knowledge (clinical)
- knowledge (non-clinical)
- skill
- attitude.

The second stage involves reflecting on these learning needs with your mentor/supervisor. These learning needs should be stimulated by the unmet patient needs that you recorded during your clinical working, compiled with other learning needs derived from other sources, such as feedback from patients or colleagues. Your learning needs may be fulfilled in a number of ways, such as by asking an experienced practitioner or by looking up what you need to know; or further study, observation of a specialist practitioner, small group discussion or other forms of learning may be required.

Producing and achieving objectives

A helpful step is to translate the learning needs into a list of objectives. When you set learning objectives try to make sure they are SMART:

SPECIFIC
MEASURABLE
ACHIEVABLE
REALISTIC
TIMEBOUND.

For example, being asked to 'improve team meetings' is not helpful unless you know how. However, being told to 'ensure all meetings have an agenda, minutes and that you keep to the allotted time' would help because you then know exactly what is expected and whether or not you have achieved the objective.

Table 5.2 contains examples of verbs that are useful when formulating objectives. For instance, 'By the end of this clinical placement I will be able to demonstrate...'

Table 5.2 Useful verbs		
Analyze	Define	Illustrate
Apply	Demonstrate	Interpret
Compare	Differentiate	List
Construct	Explain	Translate
Critique	Identify	Undertake

Reflective activity

Write an individual learning objective based on your current clinical area. Is it SMART? In what ways could you achieve this learning objective? Which learning activity best 'fits' your learning style and the skill, knowledge or attitude to be developed? What forms of evidence can you identify that could be used as the basis for assessing whether this learning outcome had been achieved?

Another way to identify your learning needs could be to undertake a SWOT analysis (Table 5.3). A SWOT analysis can be a useful tool not just for identifying individual learning needs but also for examining things that may help or hinder the learning process. You can then try to minimize anything that could impede your learning.

Table 5.3 SWOT pro forma	
Strengths	Weaknesses
Opportunities	Threats

Much of your learning is likely to be striving for clinical competence and capability.

Capability can be defined as 'everything a person can think or do, given an appropriate context for demonstrating it' (Eraut, 1998, p. 135).

Competence is the ability to perform a particular activity to a predetermined standard. This predetermined standard can be either:

- criterion referenced – based on a constant reference scale, or
- norm referenced – relating an individual's performance to that of fellow students.

Practitioners need to be able to carry out certain 'tasks' expected by their profession, and health care roles, such as nursing or physiotherapy, call for psychomotor skills as well as analytical and reflective ability. The clinical competence required for work in a practice setting is often well rooted in certain skills, but these also progress and evolve. Acceptable levels of performance influence the assessment of practice processes and also the development of tools by which to judge performance. After developing a learning objective, and agreeing a plan to achieve this, it is necessary to judge whether the learning experience has been effective; where practice skills are concerned, this is usually undertaken through an agreed set of skills criteria.

Skills criteria comprise:

1 a situation of some complexity

2 a performance that deliberately addresses the situation (not just a matter of chance)

3 an assessment that the performance has met the demands of the situation (and is supported by the existence of relevant knowledge)

4 a sense that the performance was commendable.

Undertaking competency-based assessment requires thought, analysis, staff development and effective recording. It can be concerned with what the learner does, rather than what they know, but is best applied with a mechanism that requires understanding of meaning and knowledge. It is helpful if a competency assessment tool, or practice assessment tool, has already been developed and is provided. However, if this is not the case, the learner and supervisor should agree the criteria by which the learning objective is to be judged prior to undertaking the learning activity. There is further exploration of assessment in Chapter 7.

SELF-ASSESSMENT

Self-assessment involves learners taking responsibility for monitoring and making judgements about aspects of their own learning. Although a mentor, supervisor or preceptor may be involved in assessing achievement of a learning objective, it is always useful for the learner to undertake a self-assessment. This can be informal (formative) or formal (summative) in nature and can be broken down into two stages:

1 identifying standards and/or criteria to apply to an understanding of the knowledge, skill or attitude

2 making judgements about the extent to which the learner has met these criteria and standards.

Self-assessment is increasingly being used as a formative tool in clinical education and is frequently used as a means of evaluating learning interventions. However, the ability to assess oneself is seldom tested and self-assessment skills are rarely taught. Self-assessment improves learning by developing the skills of evaluation and critical judgement. In this sense the term 'self-evaluation' may perhaps be more appropriate since it is about developing learners' ability to make judgements about the quality of their learning.

Self-assessment can:

● help learners to become critical about their own practice

● enable learners to develop their learning and assessment skills whilst engaged in practice rather than afterwards

● provide a structure for discussion about the quality of care/treatment

● help learners to understand the subjective nature of judgements in assessment and the many influences on this.

Reflective activity

Consider whether self-assessment is:

1 helpful in identifying learning needs

2 able to promote learner activity

3 likely to lead to a change in clinical practice.

THE NHS KNOWLEDGE AND SKILLS FRAMEWORK

Although individuals have different learner motivations, styles and identified learning needs, it is necessary to appreciate the requirements of a particular health care role. The NHS Knowledge and Skills Framework (KSF) has been designed as a generic development tool for use throughout the NHS to describe the knowledge and skills that are applied within health care and has been designed to support the development of staff (DoH, 2004).

Each post has a KSF outline that identifies the aspects or dimensions of knowledge and skills required for undertaking the role. The KSF is based on 30 dimensions, six core dimensions (applied in all roles) and 24 specific dimensions grouped under four themes (relevant specifically to the post) as detailed in Table 5.4.

Table 5.4   NHS Knowledge and Skills Framework
Core dimensions:
1 Communication
2 Personal and people development
3 Health, safety and security
4 Service improvement
5 Quality
6 Equality and diversity
Specific dimensions:
Promotion of Health and wellbeing (ten dimensions)
Estates and facilities (three dimensions)
Information and knowledge (three dimensions)
General (eight dimensions)

(adapted from DoH, 2004)

The NHS KSF (DoH, 2004) is designed to:

● support the effective learning and development of individuals and teams – with all staff being supported to learn throughout their careers, and being given the resources to do so

● support the development of individuals in the post in which they are employed so they can be effective at work

● promote equality for and diversity of all staff – with every member of staff using the same framework, having the same opportunities for learning and development open to them and having the same structured approach to learning, development and review.

In response to an independent enquiry, the NHS staff council (DoH, 2010b) simplified the KSF to make it easier to use and understand, the key features being focusing on the core dimensions, reducing the amount of evidence which needs to be gathered and different ways to develop outlines. A leadership and management dimension can also be included for senior management roles, stronger links identified to appraisal and the option to develop team objectives. However Trusts can still utilize the original KSF if this is helpful.

> ### ✍ *Over to you*
>
> Take a look at this website, which has been produced to inform everyone about the NHS e-KSF online tool, which supports the Knowledge and Skills Framework: **www.nhsemployers.org/PayAndContracts/AgendaForChange/KSF**

Progress towards the KSF outline should be reviewed periodically with the employee's line manager. This is usually done within a yearly appraisal. Undertaking staff appraisals may be a role requirement for individuals involved with staff development.

> **Appraisal**
> Appraisal is an organizational process for assessing the performance of staff and their requirement for learning and development. The aim of appraisal is to ensure understanding by staff of what is required of them in their role

Reflective activity

1 Think about last year – what went well and what not so well? Why was this?

2 What were the most important things that you learnt during the year?

3 Have there been changes in how you give your clinical care?

4 Have you taken on new responsibilities or seen your role change in other ways?

As explained in Table 5.5 below, the main elements of an appraisal system are:

- a review of an individual's performance
- identification of training and development needs to ensure full development within an existing post
- supporting and planning career development.

Table 5.5 Roles and responsibilities of appraiser and appraisee	
Appraisor	**Appraisee**
Understand the KSF outline for the posts that you manage or supervise	Understand the KSF outline for your post
Undertake appraisal training	Evaluate your achievements referring to the KSF outline
Undertake objective reviews of your staff's performance on a regular basis	Identify your strengths
Gather and structure evidence to show how members of staff have met their KSF outlines	Gather and structure evidence that demonstrate your achievements

(Continued)

Table 5.5 Roles and responsibilities of appraiser and appraisee (*Continued*)	
Appraisor	**Appraisee**
Alert staff to issues in their work as soon as they arise	Identify your learning and development needs
With the member of staff identify their learning and development needs ensuring that these are included in the post holder's personal development plan	Prioritize, identify and arrange training and development activities to meet your learning needs
Identify, with the appraisee, the resources – people, time, finance and equipment – to support their learning.plan	Identify your personal contribution towards your personal development plan

PERSONAL DEVELOPMENT PLANS

A personal development plan (PDP) is the outcome of a structured support process undertaken by an individual with their manager, to reflect upon their own learning, performance and achievements and to plan for their personal, educational and career development. A PDP is usually agreed through an annual meeting between the individual and their line manager where the performance and progress against the KSF outline are reviewed and new objectives agreed. Following this, there should be ongoing reviews to make sure support and learning is on track. Further information about the content and development of a personal development plan can be found in the online bonus feature that accompanies this chapter.

LEARNING CONTRACTS

There are many similarities between personal development plans and learning contracts; both are an individualized tool for promoting self-directed adult learning. Essentially, a learning contract is a written plan that describes what an individual will learn as a result of some specified learning activity. Learning contracts can take many forms and a number of terms are used interchangeably in reference to them, such as learning plans, study plans, performance agreements, or self-development plans. Learning contracts can enhance individual motivation for learning and help develop mutual respect between the mentor/supervisor and the learner.

A learning contract consists of five major elements that specify the following:

1 The knowledge, skills, attitudes and values to be acquired by the learner (learning objectives).

2 How these objectives are to be accomplished by the learner (learning resources and strategies).

3 The target date(s) for completion.

4 The evidence that will be presented to demonstrate that the objectives have been completed (evidence of accomplishment).

5 How this evidence will be judged or validated (criteria and means for validating evidence) (Knowles, 1986).

Learning contracts usually have sections for learning objectives, learning resources, evaluative evidence and how this will be verified and the associated target dates. A key to developing a successful learning contract is making the learning activities specific enough for the learner to move to action, but also sufficiently flexible to allow some individual creativity in the chosen approach. For instance, a learning need could be met through job shadowing or by participating in a project; and the individual may choose one of these as more appropriate.

Learners can be encouraged to keep a reading and evidence-base log that summarizes the theoretical learning that has been achieved whilst undertaking an activity. It needs to be stressed that the form of evidence selected when negotiating the learning contract should demonstrate accomplishment of the learning objective being pursued. If the learning contract is being undertaken as part of a formal education programme, the criteria for judging achievement are likely to be predetermined; however, if this is not the case, the final task in developing a learning contract involves determining the criteria and the means for validating and judging the evidence.

Learning contracts are inherently flexible, but perhaps because of the use of the word 'contract', with its legalistic tone, learners can get the idea that they may not change their learning contract once it has been negotiated. Renegotiations of learning contracts can occur at any time up until the end of the learning experience if plans or ideas change:

Learning contracts have a number of practical benefits:

- Learners are more involved in their own learning.

- Learning contracts help learners make use of a wide variety of resources for learning, such as peers, others in the institution and community, and field experiences.

- Learners' skills of self-directed learning are sharpened, enhancing their ability to learn from experience and from their environment for the rest of their lives.

- Learning contracts provide more functional and validated evidence of the achievement learning outcomes.

- In the learning process, the conventional mentor/supervisor-imposed discipline is replaced by self-discipline.

- Learning contracts provide a way for the learner to obtain continual feedback about progress being made toward accomplishing learning goals.

- Learning contracts are more cost-effective than traditional mentor-directed learning, in that the learner is less dependent on exclusive use of the resources of mentors/supervisors and takes some of the responsibility for directing the learning off the mentors'/supervisors' shoulders (adapted from Knowles, 1986, p. 46).

However, learning contracts have some limitations: the mentor/supervisor can encounter difficulties when taking on a more facilitative role, and it can be difficult for a learner who is very new to clinical practice to contribute towards identifying their learning needs.

KEY POINTS

Contract learning involves an agreement between at least two parties about:

● the content of the learning

● how it will be learnt

● the criteria for determining that learning has been achieved

● a diagnosis of learning needs, learning resources and strategies required

● the evidence to prove learning and a date for review of this

When implementing learning activities and evaluating learning, it may be necessary to refine the learning contract in the light of progress.

RAPID RECAP

Check your progress so far by working through each of the following questions.

1 Identify a minimum of four factors that are likely to affect an individual's learning.

2 What is a reason for finding out someone's learning style? Give the names of two models that could be used to do this.

3 What are the characteristics of information that can be used to help in the successful development of a learning objective?

4 What are the core dimensions of the NHS KSF and the role and responsibilities of an appraisee?

5 Identify the five key components of a learning contract.

If you have difficulty with any of these questions, read through the section again to refresh your understanding before moving on.

CHAPTER 6

EXPERIENTIAL LEARNING AND THE ROLE OF REFLECTION

LEARNING OBJECTIVES

By the end of this chapter you should be able to:

- define the concepts of peer learning, problem-based learning and praxis

- utilize reflective frameworks to review practice decision-making

- explore team facilitation and action learning

- value evidence-based practice and pragmatic approaches to action-planning.

Bonus features for this chapter available on the book's website

INTRODUCTION

In a single day, a health care professional has to make many rapid decisions about how to respond to unique and complex situations. This could be in relation to health care practice and service delivery or how they plan to adapt, facilitate and assess a student's learning for that shift. Yet they often seem to practise with little in the way of conscious reasoning. So how are those decisions made? Within this chapter, we will explore some of the 'scaffolding' that can help keep decisions 'on track'.

For instance, in conditions where there is too little time and many interruptions, nurses have been found to compensate by developing a range of strategies, including minimizing the time spent doing tasks, creating time and redefining the work that has to be done by prioritizing and reprioritizing (Bowers *et al.*, 2001). Nurses work at a fast pace and combine tasks (e.g. documenting a patient's fluid intake whilst watching the patient take their medication). They change the sequence of tasks (e.g. documenting care, long after its delivery), and communicate their heavy workload to patients to reduce any possible additional requests. They 'make time' by coming in early, missing meals or doing work at home (Bowers *et al.*, 2001). The underlying pattern is one of trying to maintain continuity for patients while completing as many physical tasks as possible.

In the course of this chapter, we will explore how individuals and clinical teams can work on their conscious decision-making regarding patient care. Practice involves the gaining of new knowledge by developing and applying methods that draw from situated, individual instances of practice, with practitioners critically examining practice through systematic self-reflection, reflective discourse and critically oriented change.

EXPERIENTIAL LEARNING

As professional knowledge is functioning, specific and pragmatic and deals with determining priorities and executing actions, problem-based learning appears to be a suitable method of facilitating learning. Problem-based learning starts with problems or situations rather than with the exposition of knowledge; it is sometimes called context-based learning or inquiry-based learning. Biggs (2003) considers problem-based learning to be a total approach to teaching that reflects the way that people learn in real life where they simply get on with solving the problems that life puts before them with whatever resources are to hand.

The eight tasks of problem-based learning (Wolff and Rideout, 2001) have been identified as:

1 Explore the problem, clarifying terms and concepts, creating hypotheses and identifying issues.
2 Identify what you already know that is pertinent.
3 Identify what you do not know.
4 Prioritize the learning needs, set goals and objectives, allocate resources.
5 Engage in a self-directed search for knowledge.
6 Share knowledge and information effectively with others.
7 Apply, use and explain the knowledge and skills.
8 Reflect on what has been learnt and the process of learning.

The 'coaching' approach to supervising learning in problem-based education encompasses goal setting, modelling, guiding, facilitating, monitoring, and providing feedback to learners to support their active and self-directed thinking and learning. Problem-based learning is different from conventional problem-solving learning, where the learners are set a problem or case after they have been taught the knowledge (Savin-Baden, 2000). Biggs (2003) suggests that it is important to align learning outcomes, teaching and learning activities, and assessment tasks in problem-based learning to encourage deep, rather than surface, approaches to learning.

Since Dewey (1938) argued that all learning can be viewed as experience, there is now growing consensus that experiences form the basis of learning. Professional learning, which integrates theory within practice in the workplace, challenges the curricular assumptions on which many health care programmes are based, meaning that experiential knowledge is professional practice (Richardson, 1999). One way of defining experiential learning was developed by Kolb (1984b, p. 38), who viewed this as 'the process whereby knowledge is created through the transformation of experience'. (Further discussion of Kolb's learning cycle is contained in Chapter 5.) Usher and Soloman (1999) view experiential learning as experience constructed in a particular way. This differentiation between everyday experience and experiential learning is not about devaluing experience but reinforces the need for intent in the process of learning within practice settings in order to build knowledge.

Reflective activity

Think about the key findings from the research study by Bowers *et al.* (2001) mentioned in the introduction to this chapter. Within this care home with nursing for older people, the nurses were observed to be applying a range of strategies to 'keep up' with the physical care demands of the work setting. Have you seen this happening within clinical placements? Have you been aware of using some of these strategies yourself? What role do you think reflective processes could play in exploring the effects of these strategies?

The learning cycle starts with experience, proceeds through reflection to action, which in turn becomes concrete experience for further reflection. Experiential learning can be relatively independent of organizing or mediation and takes many forms, including not only structured clinical placement experience, simulation, role-play and involvement in a change-management project but also any form of personal development. Involving others in experiential learning, for instance through action learning, allows proposed actions and their consequences to be exposed to constructive criticism.

Praxis

Praxis is a complex activity by which individuals become critically conscious human beings using a cycle of action–reflection–action that is central to learning. Characteristics of praxis include self-determination, proactive intention, creativity and conscious decision-making. Phronesis – a process of moral reasoning enacted to establish the 'good' of a particular situation and often referred to as practical wisdom – is central to the concept of praxis

(Connor, 2004). Rolfe (2006) suggests that the model in which theory is viewed as informing and controlling practice should give way to a model in which theory and practice are seen as mutually enhancing, with theory being derived from practice, and in turn influencing future practice. He refers to this coming together of theory and practice as nursing praxis, and he suggests that informal theory should be unique to each individual encounter with a patient. A clinical practitioner is also, therefore, a theorist and a researcher who responds to patients by the process of reflection-in-action, drawing upon the practitioner's expertise and a repertoire of past experiences and encounters.

KEY POINTS

● Learners are actively involved in an exploration of an experience

● Experiential learning involves a cyclical sequence of learning activities

● Learners should critically and selectively reflect on their experience

● Learners should be committed to the experiential process

● There needs to be scope for the learner to explore the experience independent from the facilitator/clinical supervisor

REFLECTION

There is a common-sense view of reflection that sees this as a way of thinking or mental processing that is done to achieve an outcome or purpose: for example, the thoughts we might have as we drive home from work, mentally reviewing the day. However, reflective learning in professional and academic contexts is likely to involve a conscious process of critical review, clarification and actions which in some instances is transformative in revising the meanings underpinning judgements.

Dewey (1938) was one of the first theorists to define reflection; he identified it as turning over in your mind a subject and giving it serious consideration. Reflection involves the movement away from acceptance of information, which novices may do, to questioning and becoming active in critically thinking and learning. Boyd and Fales (1983, p. 100) define reflection as 'the process of internally examining and exploring an issue of concern, triggered by an experience, which creates and clarifies meaning in terms of self and which results in a changed conceptual perspective'.

Reflective practice can be summarized as having three components: experience–reflection–action, termed the ERA cycle (Figure 6.1) (Jasper, 2013). These are:

1 experiences that happen to a practitioner

2 the reflective processes that allow the practitioner to learn from these experiences

3 the actions that result from the new perspectives that are achieved through reflection.

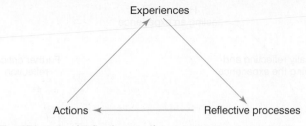

Figure 6.1   The ERA cycle of reflective practice, (adapted from Jasper, 2013)

Reflective processes include an opportunity to look at the context in alternative ways allowing us to focus on different aspects of our experiences. Cowan (1998) distinguishes between analytical and evaluative reflection: the former answers the question 'How do I do it?' and the latter 'How well can I do it?' The evaluative aspect of reflection is critical in the sense of exercising discernment and making judgements. Without such critical evaluation it would be difficult to complete the reflective process and for the learning from reflection to result in action and improvement.

Scanlon and Chernomas (1997) have suggested an alternative three-stage model of reflection:

1 awareness – initiating reflection through discomfort, lack of information or seeking an explanation

2 critical analysis – taking into account current knowledge, critically examining and thinking about the event/issue

3 new perspective – outcome of analysis and new information which leads to changes and actions/outcomes.

The connection between critical thinking and reflection is evident in much of the health care and education literature.

The process of reflection is complex and involves making a judgement on experience and making assessments in the light of a standard (either personal or drawn from others' experience). What has sometimes been omitted from a discussion of the experiential learning cycle is the need for decisions to be made. When learners systematically engage in critical thinking, they tend to develop insights into their learning processes and practice (Figure 6.2).

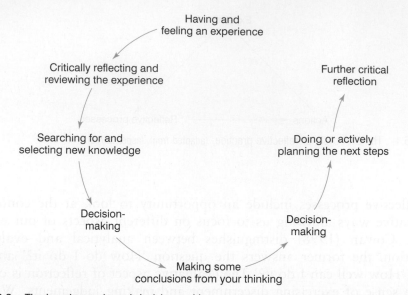

Figure 6.2   The learning cycle and decision-making, (reflects the thinking of Rogers, in Leeper, 1967)

The discussion in Chapter 5 on learning styles has made you aware of the possibility that some learners may find it difficult to think reflectively. Non-reflection is evident when a person simply mentions or describes a concept, for example, a habitual way of working, and makes no attempt to expand on this and relate it to their future working. This is termed Level 1 by Hatton and Smith (1995) who posit four levels of reflection:

1 **description** – pure description with no reflection
2 **descriptive reflection** – a description of the event; the possibility of alternative viewpoints is accepted, but mostly the reflection is from one perspective
3 **dialogic reflection** – able to step back from the event and actions and to explore and analyze these, recognizing inconsistencies and that differing judgements and alternative explanations exist
4 **critical reflection** – shows an awareness of the event and actions from multiple perspectives, understanding the influence of social and political context.

The level may affect the overall outcome of reflection, as higher-level reflection should increase clarity and personally valuable learning. Hatton and Smith's (1995) level descriptors help in encouraging students or qualified professionals to deepen their reflective skills, but you need to be aware that undertaking critical reflection requires an ability to determine an endpoint so that reflection is practical and manageable.

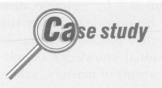

Case study

Student (community specialist practice – health visitor)

"I am at the stage when I have started to take on a supervised caseload of my own. When I came out of a 'new birth' visit to an 11-day-old baby boy and his mother, my practice teacher said she felt that the mother could be at risk of developing postnatal depression – despite the fact that she had no evidence to base this on apart from her experience and intuition. I found myself thinking, is she right, and if so will I ever feel that expert and confident?

At the next follow-up visit to this first-time mum, she appeared very happy and not as though she was suffering from classic postnatal depression. My practice teacher sat patiently and listened to the client, waiting for me to take up an opportunity to ask her about her feelings. I sat anxiously, watching what was going on and trying to work out what it all meant. Eventually, I plucked up the courage to discuss how the mother was really feeling and we filled in the Edinburgh Postnatal Depression Scale questionnaire. It became clear that the mother was relieved that we had given her an opportunity to discuss how she was feeling. She had some insight into the possibility that she may be suffering from postnatal depression and she was willing to have professional help. The mother seemed fairly comfortable with the outcome of the visit, as did my practice teacher, but this left me feeling concerned as to whether I would have been able to pick this up were I to be practising on my own as a newly qualified health visitor. Will I be able to develop the same level of expertise in recognizing postnatal depression?

As a learning experience this was very useful. I identified a deficit in my knowledge base and my practice skills. We use the Edinburgh Postnatal Depression Scale, which was developed by Cox in the 1980s for use as a screening tool. It is a self-administered questionnaire consisting of ten statements each with four possible responses, which are scored from 0 to 3 linked to perceived severity. A score of 12 or above is an indication of possible postnatal depression when combined with a clinical interview. This woman scored 13, and I now feel confident in using this to differentiate between feeling tired and tearful and suffering from postnatal depression."

What insight does this student health visitor show through this reflective account?

What level of reflection as devised by Hatton and Smith (1995) would best describe this reflective account?

What additional elements could be added to this reflection to strengthen this further?

Reference

Cox, J.L., Holden, J.M. and Sagovsky, R. (1987) Detection of postnatal depression: development of the Edinburgh Postnatal Depression Scale. *British Journal of Psychiatry*, **150**, 782–786.

Reflection often involves the highlighting of past emotional experiences. In the above case study, the student health visitor had not picked up the cues regarding possible postnatal depression but her practice teacher had, an example of the experienced practitioner knowing more than they may make explicit to a student. The expert practitioner (Schön, 1983) uses knowledge and skills influenced by attitudes to solve problems in the work place. This problem-solving process is automatic, routine and intuitive and requires little critical thinking, and has been termed reflection-in-action. Reflection-in-action is where:

- the potential range of outcomes are recognized
- the problem is reviewed and alternative hypotheses thought about
- further information is sought (either from the patient or from sources of professional knowledge, e.g. colleagues, literature).

Reflection-on-action, however, involves the situation – for example, new practice, existing practice or outmoded practice – being reviewed after the event and this leads to new learning. This retrospective process often raises questions that require further information, professional knowledge or self-inquiry. So this process adds to the development of a zone of mastery. Schön (1983) identified an interaction – in the form of synergy – between practical competence and professional artistry and hence learning.

Although professional training is based on a common knowledge or skill set, as soon as an individual engages in assessing and responding to specific patient needs, that individual's practice becomes differentiated from that of others. Practice is prevented from becoming routine owing to the uniqueness, ambiguity and potential conflict within any clinical situation. Reflection may not be an easy process to master and can be a challenge to encourage in others. Many writers have suggested strategies or frameworks for developing reflective abilities, which usually offer a series of questions or tasks to help the person advance their thinking beyond the taken for granted. This more structured approach to reflection gives time and space for thinking, what Barnett (1997) terms 'intellectual space', and also allows ownership of the learning.

Synergy
The result of two agents, forces, people or groups coming together that leads to an enhanced outcome that is greater than the sum of each part

REFLECTING ON CRITICAL INCIDENTS

Most frameworks that we will look at in the next few pages start with selecting an experience, such as an incident from practice. When a health care professional chooses an incident to reflect on, this is usually because it is significant for some reason or has a particular meaning: perhaps it is linked to an area of practice which is an identified learning need, or it relates to a difficult clinical situation where the outcome was unexpected or unwanted. Flanagan (1954) first used the term 'critical incident': such an event may be a positive or negative experience that is suitable for description in a reasonably concise way. Unfortunately, the term 'critical incident' has sometimes been misunderstood within health care, as the word 'critical' is often used to mean 'serious'. Flanagan intended 'critical' to mean something that stands out in some way. Confusion has also crept into the discussion of reflective strategies because of the idea that all stimuli for reflection come from critical incidents that have caused us uncomfortable feelings or discomfort. This is not the case: although reflection is often stimulated by unpleasant or uncomfortable feelings, much can also be gained by examining when things go well in order to build on or replicate this situation.

The stages of reflection or critical incident analysis are listed here:

- Stage 1 – selecting an experience to reflect on
- Stage 2 – describing the incident
- Stage 3 – analyzing the experience
- Stage 4 – interpreting the experience
- Stage 5 – exploring alternative perspectives on the incident
- Stage 6 – moving to action.

Reflective activity

Consider a recent experience in your own practice where you found yourself faced by a new problem or situation and were not sure about how to act. How did you reflect on the experience? What does this tell you about your use of reflective processes?

Recollections of an event change over time: closer to an event the focus is likely to be on the emotions that were displayed and the reactions to the situation; whereas, an individual may be able to think more broadly about the situation when time has elapsed. If a learner is being encouraged to discuss and reflect on a clinical incident, it can be helpful to keep written records as these allow the clinical supervisee and supervisor/mentor to revisit the records over time which is something that purely verbal reflection may not allow.

Having described the experience, the practitioner then starts to draw conclusions from what has been described and discussed. During this stage, they should be encouraged to develop a deeper understanding of the experience by exploring certain aspects of it in detail and coming to an explanation. Once an explanation has been ascertained, those involved in the reflective process can then go on to explore the alternatives.

Exploring the alternatives can be challenging, as to get the most from this part of the process the person is asked to move beyond how they have previously perceived the incident and look at different ways of understanding it. A mentor or clinical supervisor can help in offering a different way of viewing a situation, widening and deepening the learner's understanding. Identifying alternative perspectives helps the person who is reflecting to identify actions that they could take based on this new learning.

The mentor should try to make sure that the learner focuses on their own actions, weighing up the consequences of particular actions and recognizing that these must be within their sphere of control. It can be too easy just to expect others to act for them, or for others to change themselves. The mentor may also learn from this reflective activity and decide to change their ways of dealing with something as a consequence of discussing their mentee's experience. Taking action can be viewed as the final part of the reflective process, but, as reflection is cyclic, it is likely that the health care professional will undertake further reflection about the actions taken.

FRAMEWORKS FOR REFLECTION ON PRACTICE

There are many frameworks that can be used to encourage reflection on practice, and learning through reflection may be more potent if there is structure to guide the act of reflection. Some models to help you engage in the process of reflection are now discussed. There is no right one; it is important that you choose and adapt the framework that feels most comfortable for you and best assists you in learning from your experiences. Johns (2009) suggests that we should guard against using a model too prescriptively as they may appear to indicate that reflection is an orderly process, when actually it is quite complex. Initially, frameworks for reflection can be very useful, particularly to enable practitioners new to reflection to 'follow' the process through.

One well-known framework was developed by Gibbs (1988); he proposed a cycle of reflection comprising six stages and a series of cue questions to guide a practitioner through each stage of the reflective process (Figure 6.3).

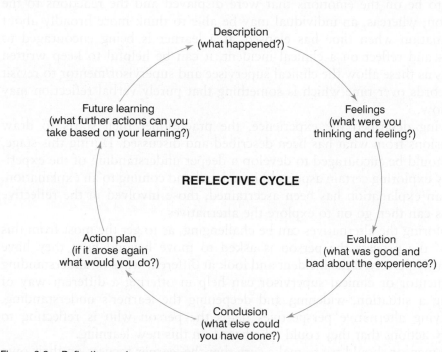

Figure 6.3   Reflective cycle, (adapted from Gibbs, 1988)

The framework devised by Palmer *et al.* (1994) also offers cues that you may find useful for structuring your reflective learning. As you will see, it is quite a simple set of questions.

REFLECTIVE FRAMEWORK

Choose and describe a situation you wish to reflect on. Ask yourself:

- What was my role in the situation?
- Did I feel comfortable or uncomfortable, why?
- What actions did I take?

- Who else was involved in the situation and how did they act?
- Were these actions appropriate?
- How could I have improved the situation for myself and others involved?
- What can I change in the future?
- Do I feel I have learnt anything new about myself?
- Did I expect anything different to happen? If yes, what?
- How has this situation changed my thinking?

(adapted from Palmer *et al.*, 1994)

Johns' (2009) structured reflection model provides a series of cue questions based on a description of the experience, reflection, influencing factors and learning. Johns has revised his reflective framework many times, incorporating Carper's (1978) 'ways of knowing', discussed previously in Chapter 2, and this is a strength of the model, which is one of the few models of reflection to refer to the development of an **epistemological** base to reflections. The cues are used as means to gain insight, with use they 'become embodied and shape the clinical gaze moment by moment in mindful attention.' (Johns, 2009, p. 51).

Epistemological
Examining the nature of knowledge and human understanding, including how knowledge is derived, determined, validated and tested

Model of structured reflection- edition 15A

Reflective cues

- Bring the mind home
- Focus on a description of an experience that seems significant in some way
- What issues are significant to pay attention to?
- How do I interpret the way people were feeling and why they felt that way?
- How was I feeling and what made me feel that way?
- What was I trying to achieve and did I respond effectively? (aesthetic)
- What were the consequences of my actions on the patient, others and myself?
- What factors influence the way I was/am feeling, thinking and responding to this situation? (personal)
- What knowledge did or might have informed me? (empirical)
- To what extent did I act for the best and in tune with my values? (ethical)
- How does this situation connect with previous experiences? (personal)
- How might I reframe the situation and respond more effectively given this situation again? (reflexivity)
- What would be the consequences of alternative actions for the patient, others and myself?
- What factors might constrain me responding in new ways?

- How do I NOW feel about this experience?
- Am I more able to support myself and others better as a consequence?
- What insights have I gained?
- Am I more able to realize desirable practice? (framing perspectives)

Johns (2009), p. 51

Additional useful information is also supplied (in Table 6.1 below) for Johns' (2000) question, 'What internal factors were influencing me?'

Table 6.1 Internal factors		
Expectations from self: – obligation/duty – conscience – beliefs/values?	Negative attitude towards the patient/family?	Expectations from others: – in what way?
Normal practice – felt I had to conform to a certain action?	What factors influenced my actions?	Loyalty to staff versus loyalty to patient/family?
Fear of sanction?	Time/priorities?	Anxious about ensuing conflict?

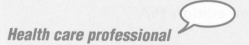

Health care professional

Registered nurse

Using reflection is something that I have always done. The important part about it for me to make it useful, is recognizing it as a continuous entity. I learn from what has gone before, appreciating that I will never encounter the same situation in exactly the same way because I have already learnt from that experience. The depth of my reflections vary, they can be relatively quick and involve decision making at that moment in time or take a much different form where I let myself explore almost all aspects of the experience looking for a deeper meaning.

Reflective activity

In the previous reflective activity within this chapter, you were asked to consider a recent experience in your own practice where you found yourself faced by a new situation. Using the cue questions from Johns' framework, write down the answers that relate to this recent experience. Then compare your learning, identified through your previous reflection, to undertaking reflection using this structured approach.

Have you gained any new insights?

Reflection helps the learner who is trying to understand meaning, but some learners may have difficulty with this way of learning and may be resistant (Boud and Walker, 1998), as their peer group's cultural norms may be more 'scientific' and this approach might be thought of as 'too woolly'.

Borton's (1970) developmental framework can assist practitioners to make sense of and then respond to real clinical situations. Borton asks the person to reflect using three basic starting points to the questions. These starting points for reflection and sample cue questions are supplied below.

Developmental framework (Borton, 1970)

1 WHAT? (Describe)

2 SO WHAT? (Theory and knowledge building)

3 NOW WHAT? (Action)

The 'what' cue questions could be, for example:

● What happened?

● What were you doing?

● What were others doing in this situation?

● What were you trying to achieve?

● What was good or bad about the experience?

The 'so what' cue questions could be, for example:

● So what additional information do I need to know in order to understand the situation?

● So what could I have done that was different?

● So what did I base my actions on?

● So what did those involved in this situation learn?

The 'now what' cue questions could be, for example:

● Now what should I do?

● Now what do I need to do to make things better?

● Now what might be the consequences of this action(s)?

● Now what contextual issues do I need to look at?

Over to you

Take a look at Jasper, M. (2013) *Beginning Reflective Practice*. 2nd edition Andover, Cengage EMEA.
   Read the section on Borton's framework and 'What? So What? Now What?' and try using the additional cue questions given for your own reflection.

Fowler (2007) has developed a linear model of reflection with options dependent on the purpose of the activity (see box below) which uses the analogy of a house. He doesn't propose that one level is more academic or better than another, they are pragmatic reflections, with each serving a specific purpose.

A linear reflective model

Factual reflection – a reflection as a photograph	Creative interpretation – reflection as modern art
The photograph is an accurate descriptive representation of the real thing. It is factual but has no interpretation, discussion or comment. It gives: ● a description of the issue or event ● the scenario ● what was its purpose ● the facts involved ● accurate description of the facts	Here the artist uses the basic structure and form of the house but this is developed and enhanced by the interpretation and interactions with other events and ideas. In this perspective, originality and alternative perspectives are dominant It is characterized by: ● discussion of alternative perspectives ● other people's perceptions of the outcome ● why things might have happened ● original ideas ● relationships and trigger factors

Creative reflection – reflection as a painting	Analytical reflection – reflection as an architect's plan
The painting starts with a fairly accurate representation of the structure and colour, etc. However, with a painting additional information is conveyed, that of emotion and feelings. The artist is interpreting the house and its environment and communicating those feelings to the person viewing the painting. This type of reflection encompasses: ● conveying the facts ● how I felt about it ● how others responded to my actions ● what I felt was important ● my perception of the outcome ● how I identified priorities.	This is the view of the house as a series of architect's plans, containing details of the structure, building materials, specifications for the size and fittings etc. It also contains details of the regulations regarding type of building materials and planning plus health and safety issues, Reflection focuses on: ● interrelationships of one part or another ● outside influences and/or regulations ● logical structure that others can follow ● well thought out over a period of time ● long term consequences ● cognisance of the environment into which it will fit.

(Fowler, 2007, p. 889)

Problems encountered when using reflection as the basis for learning are usually due to inexperience or misunderstanding. For example, when models of reflection are used as checklists for learners to work through in a methodical manner without any regard to their personal issues, there is a risk that reflection becomes ritualized and 'recipe following' (Boud and Walker, 1998). Facilitators of reflection need to be aware that reflection leads to serious questioning, and this means not only that it cannot be contained within a 'comfort zone' but also that it can foster a critical approach to understanding the clinical context. Reflection can also become rather intellectualized, with feelings and emotions being denied or lessened. Trusting others with our reflections inevitably involves risk, and enabling enough trust for emotional disclosure creates challenges for all involved. When facilitating reflection we may make assumptions about a particular event (Boud and Walker, 1998), and it can be taxing to respect learners and their agendas and take these as the focus rather than the agendas of the clinical placement area. Despite this, reflective processes are crucial to experiential learning and are something worth working on.

KEY POINTS

- Build on the way you reflect already. Try becoming more aware of how, when and why you reflect on things

- Put time aside to reflect on a regular basis, and take up opportunities to share your reflection with others, e.g. your clinical supervisor

- Try using a structured approach, e.g. a framework with cue questions, as a starting point for developing your own methods

- If you keep your own 'reflective journal or diary', read over the entries on a regular basis and look for themes

- Consider how far you are reaching any goals or taking actions you set yourself as part of reflecting

- Look for changes in yourself, your actions, attitudes, confidence and practice

- Notice and celebrate your achievements

- Be positive about the process: it takes time for progress to be made, but you will see the benefits of reflection over time

ACTION LEARNING

Action learning involves the application of the experiential learning cycle to work activities; it is linked to action research and structured reflection and shares the same processes. Action learning aims to help individuals and teams free themselves from any oppressive structures and taken-for-granted aspects about their everyday practice (Manley *et al.*, 2005) and builds on the strengths of students and staff by using a solution-focused approach.

Action learning involves five stages:

1 Reflect on current working.
2 Develop a plan of action to improve what is already happening.
3 Implement the plan.
4 Observe the effects of the action.
5 Reflect on these effects as a basis for future action planning.

There is, therefore, a continuing cycle of improvement based on evidence, in its broadest sense, and the practicalities of the clinical setting. The starting point for a cycle of action learning might be an observation of a problem in your own clinical setting. For example, a nurse might notice that the two teams delivering care on a ward often have varying workloads, and some people within the team feel overloaded. Some reflection on this problem might lead to the analysis that responsibilities have not been divided up appropriately or that the geographical divisions of patient care within the team need to be reconsidered. An action plan might involve changing some individuals' responsibilities or a change in the patient assignment method for the two teams. The ward staff could then operate for a specified time period with the new responsibilities/patient allocations, during which time the effect on workloads, team morale and delays in getting jobs done could be monitored. At the end of the trial period, all team members could contribute through reporting back as to whether the change in practice has been beneficial. This action learning cycle could lead to a new understanding of how to share the work more effectively within the ward.

An action learning team (often termed 'set') is based on the relationships between individuals in the group and they then plan future action within the structured attention and support of the group. Put simply, action learning is about solving real problems and getting things done, and it can be a method of personal management and organizational development.

Reflective activity

What possible anxieties or concerns would you have, if your clinical team decided to use action learning as a method of working on improvements in the clinical setting?

It is important to have **empathy** with participants in action learning sets who have a 'problem'. It is useful to cultivate an attitude that is curious and thoughtful about the way the person feels about the problem under discussion. This enables participants to be more open about their problem, and, in being so, they discover issues of which they were themselves previously unaware.

It is usually the case that each person in a set would have a slightly different reaction if they were in the same situation. For this reason, it can be unhelpful to describe 'what I would do in your situation'. One way to approach this is simply to ask 'How do you feel about...?' The answers are often surprising and help the participant to recognize their own feelings about an issue.

Action learning is a method that helps participants to develop by learning from each other, and it is a structured way of tackling everyday problems in a supportive yet challenging and informed way. The method requires team members to come together on a regular basis to share their problems and experiences. There are usually three stages: identifying and clarifying the problem, listing possible actions, and selecting which specific action to take. Although there may be team 'problems' to tackle, members of an action learning set retain responsibility for working on and solving their own problems.

Empathy
The willingness to share and understand another person's feelings and thoughts, so that you can help them to solve their own problem. Cultivating empathy, the ability to appreciate and believe how it feels to be in another's shoes, leads to more trusting relationships

Health care professional

Action learning participant

This was the first time I had been involved in action learning, although I have obviously worked in many group or team situations before. I hadn't thought about how much I enjoyed it until we came to the end of the project. I reflected on why I had enjoyed this particular group work so much. Part of it was because the group members were very dedicated to the group and really easy to get along with. I now see that it was also more related to the fact that we spent quite a time early on in group-building functions, such as the development of ground rules. We also worked on maintaining the group, by keeping notes and holding people to agreed actions. I now realize there was a lot of co-ordinating, facilitating, supporting and encouraging going on. This has made me consider how I will set up future team meetings and group working.

If members of a clinical team work together as an 'action learning set', they can start to improve their performance by taking action and then reviewing their results. Sometimes, a facilitator can help others in learning about key problems within everyday experience and by reviewing progress. Whilst planning and initiating team or care delivery changes, set participants also have an opportunity to review their own development needs and try out personal changes. As a result, set participants improve their own and their organization's performance. Action learning sets can enable participants to make commitments to action that they would not necessarily be in a position to take as an individual working in isolation or just from having listened to a lecture or seminar. Action learning sets help with the management of change and the development of leadership skills (see Table 6.2).

Table 6.2 Benefits of action learning	
Individual practitioner	**Organization/clinical area**
Greater breadth in understanding their organization and building relationships necessary to take action	Shared knowledge and learning from wider range of colleagues.
More ability to analyze ambiguous data and solve complex problems	Enables effective action to be taken to creatively resolve difficult problems, to do things differently and improve continuously
Enhanced capacity to understand and initiate organizational changes	Organizational/clinical care change required as well as personal change
Increased focus on what makes a difference in a situation	More likely to develop leaders with a flexible, entrepreneurial approach (at all levels) who can manage change and uncertainty

(Continued)

Table 6.2 Benefits of action learning (*Continued*)	
Individual practitioner	**Organization/clinical area**
Being more action focused and proactive in delivering results	Able to tackle difficult problems or when the organization/clinical area faces crises, improving morale
Enhanced self-awareness and appreciation of personal impact on others, contributing to improved ability to work with others in teams	More cost effective than 'traditional' training courses and intimately linked to organization/clinical area working
Developed flexibility in responding to changing situations and adapting a more flexible range of behaviour	Encourages effective teamwork, focuses and sustains the motivation of committed people and co-operation across internal organizational boundaries
Greater effectiveness in communicating proposals to senior managers	Offers an integrated path to personal and organizational learning at as fast a rate as the changes in the outside world

Organizing the meetings for an action learning set

The first task of an action learning set is to agree the ground rules. Examples of a few ground rules for one action learning set are shown here.

Examples of ground rules for an action learning set

- All group members to agree that all discussions within the action learning set should remain confidential.
- If something is discussed that an action-set member feels that they will have to take outside of the set (e.g. a code of conduct issue), this should be done with the agreement of the group.
- All group members should be supportive to each other, as well as willing to challenge.
- All participants should listen without interrupting and should actively listen, with no 'side-talking'.
- There is no such thing as a 'stupid' question.
- Make it fun.
- These ground rules are to be referred to at the beginning of each meeting and are subject to revision by the group.

Relationships are built up over time, and members care about projects succeeding. Either the facilitator or the group or both will agree how time available for the meeting will be divided so that each member gets a share of the time to focus on their own learning, or to contribute to a shared project. The action learning set looks at each issue in turn, analyzing it using a critical incident/reflective process framework. Any actions identified should be recorded so that progress can be monitored. It is also useful if a record is made of key elements of the discussion; tasks and activities to be undertaken can then be signed up to in the form of an action plan.

Depending on the nature of the problem or project and the time scales, the action learning set will meet regularly with their facilitator, at mutually agreed times, dates and places, normally for around half a day. The set participants review progress, present recommendations, agree courses of action and evaluate results. There may be some shared preparation work to do between meetings. Everyone needs to honour these commitments if the set is to function effectively and complete its tasks.

Johnson and Johnson (1992) suggest that an effective co-operative learning group should contain five critical elements:

- positive interdependence – the trust among members that holds the group together
- interpersonal social skills – the ability to communicate with each other effectively
- reflection on group functioning and feeding this back to each other
- exchange of ideas and resources, promoting higher-level decision-making
- individual accountability, with all contributing to group accountability.

There is a constant and fascinating tension between the organizing ability and facilitation skills of an outside facilitator and the team or community with which they are working. The facilitator is always in danger of 'helping' in a way that is not helpful because it is too controlling or because they fail to understand the situation, because they are an 'outsider'. The community is always in danger of irrationally rejecting the outsider or of becoming overly dependent. For these reasons, facilitators of action learning must follow frameworks for reflective practice and carefully monitor their facilitation practices (Kristiansen and Bloch-Poulsen, 2004).

It can be helpful if participants in an action-learning set prepare for set meetings by reading through their notes and recording their progress towards their action points beforehand. The set might agree to more elaborate forms of preparation, such as sending round forms with a synopsis of the work done since the last meeting. The group may invite brainstorming or force field analysis (factors hindering or facilitating a particular action plan) from the group, or present progress by a flipchart or handout, or simply hold an unstructured discussion. The following pro forma may be useful in aiding documentation.

Action Learning Set pro forma: Status report

Date .... Time ....

What actions have I completed since the last meeting?
Action points outstanding:
What were the outcomes?
What is/are my most pressing problem(s)?
What do I want to achieve by the next meeting? Proposed next steps:
What could get in the way of achieving the next steps?
What do I want to get from the meeting?
Reflections of the meeting/feedback from group members:

KEY POINTS

- Successful action-learning groups call for non-judgemental attitudes, not imposing one's views or attitudes, asking questions rather than giving advice, and respecting the view of others.

- Action learning combines learning by taking action on real problems with learning from reflective self-assessment and review. Participants learn by diagnosing problems and devising solutions but also by making decisions and being responsible for achieving outcomes.

- Action learning sets often tackle crucial organizational problems for which there are no known answers. This involves participants moving beyond comfortable, familiar tasks to focus on how they respond to challenging, unfamiliar problems and will support innovation.

- Participants volunteer to tackle important problems that they want to have impact on and are willing to commit their time, energy and capabilities to resolving.

- Action learning focuses not only on how to tackle problems but also on the participant's own behaviour; strengths and development needs.

- Action learning offers opportunities to develop effective ways of working together and focus on teamwork and networking as well as the tasks.

- A facilitator can create the structure, process and the conditions for learning; providing both support and challenge; encouraging open feedback, questioning and encouraging exchanges of ideas or experiences. A facilitator can also provide a vital outside perspective on projects and personal development.

- Participants meet regularly during an agreed period of time to review progress and proposals to tackle difficulties, as well as to review their own learning, perceptions, behaviour and attitudes.

PEER LEARNING

Peer learning involves peers learning from each other, and action-learning sets offer one method of encouraging peer learning. All of the people involved in peer learning should be equally dedicated to helping each other. For peer learning to be effective, the group needs to experience 'positive interdependence' (emphasizing the importance and uniqueness of each person's efforts), face-to-face interaction and ensure that individual and group accountability are maintained.

Reflective activity

What experiences have you had in relation to peer learning? If it was successful think about why this was so. If it was not helpful, why was this?

How could you introduce peer learning into your current continuous professional development activities?

Peer learning extends beyond the task or project to develop leadership and relationship skills. Peer learning may, however, if poorly constructed, allow some team members to avoid fulfilling their team responsibilities. If the peer learning is part of the summative assessment, this particular problem, of individuals not taking on a suitable level of individual responsibility, can be minimized by including peer assessment of the individual performance of team members, as well as giving the group an overall assessment result. By asking for feedback from a peer, practitioners can learn about aspects of their practice of which they may not have been aware. Peer feedback can also build on self-assessment by providing greater awareness of strengths and opportunities for learning.

KEY POINTS

- Discuss incidents or examples from practice that illustrate your learning needs
- Ask peers to identify things that you do well in your practice as well as things that could enhance your practice
- Combine feedback from peers with your own self-assessment
- Choose peers who are familiar with your area of practice
- A peer does not have to come from the same professional group
- You can choose more than one peer to give you feedback
- A peer does not have to observe a practitioner's practice directly to be able to provide constructive feedback

DECISION-MAKING AND ACTION PLANNING

Action and peer learning often take the form of working individually or together on a 'project'. A project can provide an important locus for learning (DeFillippi, 2001). Project work frequently leads participants along a 'journey through practice', where knowledge can be changed, shared, discarded or embedded. The article cited in the following Evidence base provides an example of a clinical setting undertaking action learning to bring about improvements in care.

EVIDENCE BASE

Take a look at Hewison *et al.* (2011) Leading end of life care: an action learning set approach in nursing homes. *International Journal of Palliative Nursing*, **17**(3): 135–141.

In this article Hewison and her colleagues report how learning as a result of action learning enables staff to develop improvements which included more consistent use of care plans, more training for staff and increased involvement for clients and their families in planning care.

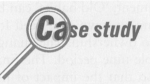

Knowledge underpinning practice decisions

Alex, an oncology specialist nurse, had to explain the various choices open to the woman with breast cancer. Alex wanted to know whether she had really done her best for the patient, so that the woman was fully informed prior to making her treatment decision.

Alex started to think about what had influenced her approach to patient communication. She had sat down with the patient and discussed the various oncology treatment options and had given the woman some information leaflets to take away to help her think things through. She had also given her contact telephone numbers so that, if the patient had any further points that needed clarifying, she could phone and ask. From past experience, Alex has come to see that patients understand and cope better with chemotherapy when they have it explained in this way. Various ways of explaining chemotherapy, including discussion alone, videos and the stories of other patients, had been tried previously, but, through 'trial and error' and watching other expert nurses in her past clinical working life, she determined that verbal discussion backed up with information leaflets was the 'best' approach. Based on what she felt intuitively would work with a particular patient and on non-verbal cues that she picked up, the way that Alex talked to each woman was different (not in content but style). Alex was also aware, through her post-registration studies, that the combination of verbal and written information leads to increased retention of the information and that patients informed in this way experience significantly less anxiety. Alex also made sure that she had the current evidence base, regarding the treatment regimens on offer, and had sought updating from journals and from other colleagues regarding the drugs available; she was also aware of her NHS Trust hospital's drug protocols for patients with this form of breast cancer.

Having read Alex's case study, identify the underlying reasons or 'source of knowledge' that she used to make her clinical decision.

Do you have any thoughts about her clinical reasoning?

Evidence-based practice

In order to approach clinical decision-making in an 'evidence-based' way, you need to review the evidence available, thinking carefully and clearly about what makes most sense in influencing your clinical decisions. Evidence-based practice means integrating individual clinical expertise with the best available external evidence. There are advantages for health care professionals who practice in an evidence-based way as it means that their knowledge base continues improving and that they have increased confidence in their clinical decision-making. Research needs to be relevant to the clinical situation, acceptable to the professional and the patient, comprehensive, accurate, easily accessible, and understandable if nurses and other health care professionals are to implement the findings (Walsh and Wigens, 2003).

Evidence-based practice is a total process, which begins with knowing what clinical questions to ask and searching for relevant literature. Once all the relevant literature has been read and critically examined, this is shared and discussed with other clinical team members to find out whether they think it is relevant to practice. A comparison needs to be made between the 'best practice' identified through the literature search and the practice that currently exists, and thought given as to whether this 'best practice' is appropriate to the clinical setting. The evidence may support the previous practice, or there may be a need for change management. 'Old habits' can be hard to break so it is necessary for the whole team to 'own' the need for change, and action learning can be a useful route to ownership. The change needs to be maintained in practice over a reasonable time period. The final aspect of the process is the collation of evidence so that the impact of the change to practice can be assessed and evaluated (Walsh and Wigens, 2003).

Stages in the evidence-based practice process

1 Identify an area of practice.
2 Undertake a literature review.
3 Discuss the available literature with colleagues.
4 Agree 'best practice' with colleagues.
5 Compare 'best practice' to current practice.
6 Make a change in practice if necessary.
7 Evaluate the new practice.

Whatever the scenario, effective action planning involves:

• breaking your goals down into smaller steps
• identifying the actions you need to take for each step

- considering how to overcome any constraints
- identifying people/resources that can help
- setting a target date for completion of each step
- trying to be realistic in the tasks you set yourself
- monitoring, reviewing and adapting the action plan on a regular basis.

Over to you

Think about a recent area of your practice where you or your clinical team had to action plan.
Ask yourself the following questions:

1 What result was I/were we trying to achieve?
2 What activities did I/we plan in order to achieve it?
3 Did I/we achieve the planned result?
4 If not, why not?
5 Did the activities make sense, in terms of what I/we were trying to achieve?
6 Could I/we have achieved the same result at less cost, spending less time, using fewer resources, with less strain on the people involved?
7 What would I/we do differently in future?
8 What have I learnt from this analysis?

When making a change in practice it is useful to have baseline information about the current practice to allow comparison when actions are taken, but do not just collect information for the sake of having it. You must have a purpose and a reason for collecting the information, particularly if other practitioners will be required to expend effort to help in the data collection. You need to focus your information-collection process around the questions that you want answered. Usually, when you are looking for evidence, it is to show progress in activities and to allow later comparison of efficiency, effectiveness and impact.

At the start of action planning, the questions to ask include:

- What sort of information do we need?
- How will we use the information?
- How can it be collected with the least possible trouble?
- Who will collect it?

- Who will analyze it?
- At the end of the delivery of the action plan, evaluation questions you might want to answer are:

  - How many?
  - How well?
  - How often?
  - Who benefited?
  - How did they benefit?

When you analyze the information, you are looking for the unexpected, and trying to learn from any deviations (differences from the expected) so that you can improve your practice.

Monitoring an action plan requires ongoing assessment of progress and can be done by the individuals involved, or people external to delivering the change can be asked to monitor progress: for example, a manager who is a stakeholder. Monitoring progress against action learning plans enables you to learn from mistakes and take corrective action when necessary. Once the goals of the action plan have been achieved, it is useful to evaluate the overall action planning process to identify learning.

KEY POINTS

- Many different forms of evidence can be used to inform clinical decisions and actions
- Effective action planning involves breaking down goals into smaller steps and considering how these can best be achieved
- It is useful to determine and collect baseline information prior to making a change to practice, so that, after the change has been implemented and when relevant information is collected, this can determine efficacy

PROFESSIONAL PORTFOLIOS

The professional portfolio is considered to be one medium for expressing expertise, critical thinking and the progression from novice to expert. Health care professionals have to provide evidence of their competence and professional development to patients, their statutory bodies and their employer. A professional portfolio is a collection of individual material, providing proof of personal growth, continuing professional development, lifelong learning and competence. A profile is a public version of the portfolio that summarizes the content of the professional portfolio and can be submitted to professional bodies as proof of continuing professional development, or be used within an application for a position (Pearce, 2003).

All nurses and midwives on the professional register need to maintain a personal professional profile (Nursing and Midwifery Council, 2011a). If a nurse or midwife wants to retain registration they have to provide evidence within their personal professional profile that they have spent at least five days (35 hours) within the previous three years updating their knowledge and skills (Nursing and Midwifery Council, 2011a). Practitioners also need to have completed a minimum of 60 days (450 hours) of practice during the last three years to renew their registration.

The NMC calls it a personal professional profile and states that it is a record of career progress and professional development. The Health Professions Council (HPC) calls it a profile and uses it to demonstrate CPD and lifelong learning. The HPC (2011) states registered practitioners must:

- maintain a continuous, up-to-date and accurate record of their CPD activities;
- demonstrate that their CPD activities are a mixture of learning activities relevant to current or future practice;
- seek to ensure that their CPD has contributed to the quality of their practice and service delivery;
- seek to ensure that their CPD benefits the service user; and upon request, present a written profile (which must be their own work and supported by evidence) explaining how they have met the standards for CPD.

The HPC also links renewal of registration with evidence of continuing professional development, and revised CPD rules have been implemented (Health Professions Council, 2011). The HPC does not specify and monitor the number of hours of each registrant or number of study sessions attended, as there is a wish to be flexible to encompass the differing professional groups. Registrants are required to maintain a record of CPD activity and to make a self-declaration of their compliance to CPD standards. The Governing Council can ask at any time for a registrant to submit their CPD summary of recent work and practice as a profile. A *pro forma* is provided for the profile, and documentary evidence to support this needs to be available if required.

An effective portfolio is a visual representation of a practitioner's experience, strengths, abilities and skills. Cross-referencing, editing and imaginative paper management are important competencies in portfolio compilation. Recently, there has been general movement in portfolio development towards electronic portfolios, as these make use of current technology and can also allow for more creative and flexible visual records (Barrett, 2002). Further guidance on how to structure and develop a CPD portfolio can be found as a bonus feature in the accompanying online resources for this chapter.

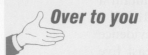

Over to you

Review your portfolio of practice:

- Is it in an easily understandable format for someone to read?
- Does it present an accurate picture of your current level of practice?
- What do your reflections cover? (Reflections should not all be on issues of concern but rather offer a more balanced evaluation of the individual practitioner's abilities and potential.)
- Does your portfolio include evaluations of successful development to date?
- Identify what you could add or need to do to improve your portfolio.

This chapter has provided you with an understanding of a number of concepts that are related to experiential learning, such as peer, problem-based and action learning. As the discussion and examples of frameworks have shown, reflective practice can facilitate clinical decision-making, and the use of a range of evidence to inform practice is encouraged. We hope this chapter has provided you with some practical ways of starting reflective practice on your own, in pairs, or within groups.

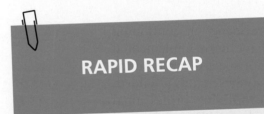

RAPID RECAP

Check your progress so far by working through each of the following questions.

1 How does experiential learning differ from classroom-based traditional teaching?

2 List three frameworks that can guide reflection.

3 What are the stages of the adapted Gibbs' reflective cycle?

4 What stages are there in making an evidence-based change in practice?

5 Can you identify the components of a professional portfolio/profile.?

If you have difficulty with any of these questions, read through the section again to refresh your understanding before moving on.

CHAPTER 7

FOCUSING ON ASSESSMENT

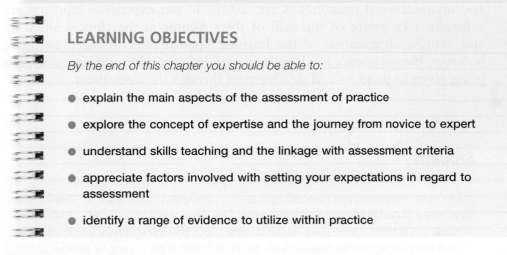

LEARNING OBJECTIVES

By the end of this chapter you should be able to:

- explain the main aspects of the assessment of practice

- explore the concept of expertise and the journey from novice to expert

- understand skills teaching and the linkage with assessment criteria

- appreciate factors involved with setting your expectations in regard to assessment

- identify a range of evidence to utilize within practice

Bonus features for this chapter available on the book's website

INTRODUCTION

Assessing another health care practitioner's practice is a privilege, and the learner is also privileged to receive the time and effort given to their assessment by a more experienced practitioner. To get the most from assessment, learners need to feel able to discuss their learning needs and be open to constructive feedback in the work setting. Much of the literature on the assessment of practice is concerned with what students should be learning and how to measure it. If the teaching methods used are experiential and focus on emulating professional practice, it is essential that practice assessment should be performance based, holistic, and allow learners to input their own decisions and solutions (Biggs, 2003). Anecdotal evidence suggests that students are assessment driven and courses can be perceived as assessment 'heavy'. The approach and attention to this varies, with some students focusing on 'getting skills signed off' rather than benefitting from a wider learning experience. Wellard *et al.* (2007) describe nursing as a practice based discipline that is dependent on being able to demonstrate competence in clinical practice, with this assessment of competence being long established (Wallace, 2003). The NMC (2008) states that the mentor must be competent to assess learning.

Assessment of practice, it is argued, should encourage critical thinking, reflective practice and skills based on sound clinical knowledge. It also provides the opportunity to nurture and develop the student's confidence as a practitioner (Aston and Hallum, 2011).

Within this chapter we will take a look at practice assessment and the evidence that can be used to demonstrate that standards are being met. As portfolio-based continuous assessment is the most commonly used format, this will also be discussed. Novices increase their expertise through working in practice, and this is also addressed.

It is important to remember that nursing draws on multiple forms of knowledge, and development is influenced by the practice context, culture and organizational structures (Carr, 2005). In our experience students are generally very aware of the skill of their mentor in the clinical situation and express appreciation of the learning opportunities afforded to them; however, the experience needs to be a rounded one, with sufficient attention being given to progress and development through the assessment.

Student

I was quite concerned that I wouldn't get all of my competencies signed off. There were only a few shifts left to work with my mentor. The assessment dictated what I learnt on the ward... at times. I even gave up the chance of going to the endoscopy unit with one of the patients to observe a procedure, because it was not a priority to achieve in my assessment of practice learning outcomes.

ASSESSMENT OF PRACTICE

Learning in practice accounts for a significant amount of time in pre-registration courses due to the very nature of health care practitioner roles. At least 50 per cent of all programmes are assessed directly in practice. Anecdotal evidence and local experience suggests that assessors in practice find this role challenging and express difficulty in interpreting assessment criteria. This is supported by the literature (Finnerty et al., 2006; Hyatt et al., 2008).

All stakeholders need be assured of the quality of assessment in practice. This supports the fundamental tenet that by the end of the programme students will be appropriately deemed as fit for purpose and practice. This is by virtue of accurate judgements derived from effective assessment which is underpinned by robust processes.

There are several strands to the context of assessment in practice (Figure 7.1), they concern all aspects of assessment.

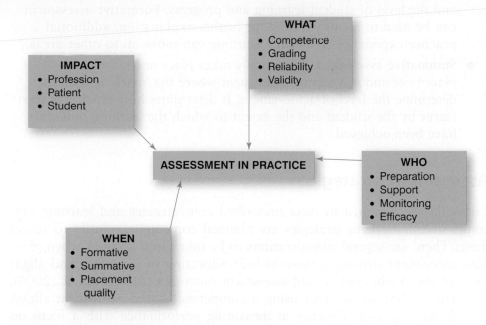

Figure 7.1   Factors impacting on assessment in practice

According to Walsh (2010) students' clinical practice is assessed for a variety of reasons, these include: monitoring progress; giving feedback; uncovering learning needs; motivating students; assessing levels of competence; assessing knowledge, skills and attitude; measuring effectiveness of teaching and always safeguarding the patient and protecting the public. In reality the definition of assessment depends on what we are assessing as well as why we are assessing (Walsh, 2010). Ultimately the aim of competency-based assessments is to produce nurses who deliver high quality care (Dolan, 2003). Professional bodies, professional education providers and the government, all have an influence over what this 'competence' is (Eraut, 1998).

Separating assessment into 'assessment of theory' and 'assessment of practice' is artificial and does not help the student practitioner. Contemporary assessment encompasses practice and theory, as well as summative and formative elements, and this is often facilitated through learning contracts and personal portfolios (Jasper, 1996). Put simply, assessment consists of finding out what and how much a person has learnt. There has been growing concern about the competence of health care professionals and the need to assess discrete skills, and this has led to the relocation of assessment into practice areas with clinical staff involvement. Assessment in practice encompasses a range of methods to measure a learner's competence to practise clinical skills and gives an assessor an opportunity to provide feedback, support and guidance.

Assessment is usually categorized as either formative or summative.

- **Formative assessment** This takes place throughout the placement and is an informal assessment that helps to identify strengths and weaknesses and the level of student learning and progress. Formative assessment can be used to identify a need for further explanation, additional practice experience or whether learning can move on to other areas.

- **Summative assessment** This usually takes place at the end of a placement and is a formal assessment where the 'mark' is used to determine the level of achievement. It determines how much has been learnt by the student and the extent to which the learning outcomes have been achieved.

Assessment strategies

Curricula are designed to meet prescribed competencies and learning outcomes and assessment strategies are planned contemporaneously to reflect these. There are several considerations to be taken into account when planning assessment strategies; these include allocation of resources and alignment of the taught content and assessment outcomes (Morgan *et al.*, 2004). Fordham (2005) advises that using a competency-based assessment allows for adaptability and efficiency in measuring performance with a focus on outcomes.

Assessment strategies contain various tools to help mentors differentiate between levels of performance and this strengthens the ability to discriminate when assessing (Aston and Hallum, 2011). Pre-registration nursing courses have a competency-based practice element, with performance being judged in line with pre-determined assessment criteria. Whilst mentoring skills continue to develop with each student, assessing skills need to be effective from the first day of mentoring (Aston and Hallum, 2011).

Continuous assessment of practice is seen as being more representative than 'one-off' assessment, where factors such as ill health and anxiety can adversely affect the outcome. Continuous assessment through portfolio assessment is more likely to motivate deep learning (Tiwari and Tang, 2003) and can include evidence of the demonstration of skills and knowledge in practice, an analysis of a critical incident, or a reflection on actual practice. However, continuous assessment takes time and energy, and protected time should be allocated and prioritized for 'assessment-only' activities (Phillips *et al.*, 2000b). Portfolio assessment also allows for the existence of unintended learning (Biggs, 2003). McMullan *et al.* (2003) suggest that portfolio assessment should contain a case made by the learner as to how the prescribed outcomes have been attained, and evidence should be offered to support this case.

However, if not approached correctly, continuous assessment can become a one-off assessment, which then reduces the predictive validity (Aston and Hallum, 2011). Assessment through observation in the work place is authentic, and interferes less with the ongoing service commitment of qualified staff (Simons and Parry-Crooke, 2001). Judgements regarding student competency are best made through observation, while standing nearby or a short distance away (Ohrling and Hallberg, 2001b). When students undertake complex tasks, they can be provided with hints before, during or after these interventions from their mentors, but, if an emergency situation occurs, the student should step back to allow the experienced practitioner to lead on care (Ohrling and Hallberg, 2001b). Previous clinical incidents can be discussed, and reflection on this, when combined with observation, is viewed as optimum for accurate assessment of practice.

Assessment responsibilities

Mentors and assessors have the following responsibilities regarding assessment:

- to maintain high personal standards of practice, teaching and assessment
- to determine the standard of care delivery of learners, and to make professional judgements about student performance from this
- to actively contribute to what is taught, learnt and assessed within clinical practice.

When student learning is taking place, the mentor is responsible for ensuring that preparation is sufficient not to put patients at risk, and that confidentiality is maintained within any documentation contained in assessment portfolios. Valid assessment can be put at risk if the mentor's role as a confidence-builder is given precedence over giving unfavourable feedback. A degree of self-reported working by a student or testimonial evidence is acceptable, but this should not form the main basis of the overall assessment decision. Practitioners who have been adequately prepared for the assessment role should have confidence in their individual assessment judgements, in the same way that they make confident decisions about client care. As students move through different clinical placements they are being assessed by many practitioners and, collectively, this process should reduce concerns about the overall subjectivity of the assessment process for a student on a registered professional course.

Mentors need to be confident in the grounding of their practice, recognize the basis of their expectations and then apply this consistently. Any assessment strategy should be able to be scrutinized in terms of objectivity (Dolan, 2003), however in reality clinical assessments do rely on the potentially subjective judgement of one mentor. Watson *et al.* (2002) view the assessment of clinical competence as challenging. Facing decisions around what and how an objective assessment can really take place is a dilemma for educators and some mentors, however many mentors give this concept little thought on an everyday level. Mentors are primarily concerned with carrying out their role as health care professionals, and therefore may not have much time to think about the objectivity of their assessment of their mentee.

In their study, Bray and Nettleton (2007) identified that assessment was identified as less of a priority than the more pastoral aspects of mentorship, adding that the poor recognition of the formal assessor role is of concern. It is widely acknowledged that mentors face competing priorities and constraints (Phillips *et al.*, 2000b; Edmond, 2001; Fordham, 2005; Kilcullen, 2007; Myall *et al.*, 2008). This has not changed over the last decade. Assessors utilize their own unrecognized time in order to reflect and prepare feedback (Malik and McGowan, 2007).

The more experienced the assessor, the more they will have internalized a model of competence which in turn affects the degrees of judgemental aggregation: this means to compensate, make allowances, interpret, and explain away situations (Stuart, 2007). On the other hand, the inexperienced practitioner/assessor does not make as many allowances or compensations; they expect every performance criteria to be achieved (Stuart, 2007).

Nurses can overlook the complexity of the interaction and skill required to perform in a clinical context as they develop professionally, as once this is internalized it becomes automatic and is not easy to articulate (Edmond, 2001) As a result this skill is not always used to the full potential in teaching or assessment. Stuart (2007) reminds us that the point is not that assessors cannot assess to an acceptably common standard: they can; however, the process is complex and judgemental. The use of a clinical assessment schedule which could assist with conscious assessment, giving the learner the opportunity to practice, receive feedback and progress, could form the structure and detail to focus on each week (Price, 2007) Aston and Hallum (2011) suggest using the everyday skills you possess for practice, planning and organizing, in assessing the student's progress, and trying not to leave it until the last minute.

NOVICE TO EXPERT

Assessing practice evidence can help in determining the level of practice working. Benner (1984) identified the 'journey' that students take from being novices (students) to expert practitioners, and how nurses uncover and create knowledge through actual experiences. She built on the work of Dreyfus and Dreyfus (1979) and their model of skill acquisition developed through researching trainee aircraft pilots, which produced five levels of proficiency in the movement of novice to expert. Benner (1984) interviewed beginning nurses and expert nurses who had both been involved in the same situations, and examined both forms of narrative. An interpretative approach was then used to analyze the data, taking into account the context and the meaning that they made of the situation. Benner found that the key to expert practice was the ability to 'experience nursing' and then to integrate this into existing and new knowledge. The five levels of proficiency identified by Benner are outlined here.

Levels of proficiency (after Benner, 1984)

1 **Novice** – have had no experience of the situation; may show rigid adherence to taught rules and plans, little situational perception, no discretionary judgement

2 **Advanced Beginner** – demonstrates marginally acceptable performance, using guidelines for action, based on attributes or aspects; situational perceptions still limited; all attributes and aspects are treated separately and given equal importance

3 **Competent** – has been in similar situations and begins to see his or her actions in terms of the 'bigger' picture; coping with many forms of information, sees actions partly in terms of long-term goals, conscious planning, standardized and routinized procedures

4 **Proficient** – perceives situations as a whole and demonstrates a 'smooth' clinical performance; sees what is most important in a situation, perceives deviations from the normal, decision-making less laboured

5 **Expert** – no longer relying on principles, rules or guidelines to connect their actions to the appropriate situation; intuitive grasp of situations based on tacit understanding, analytical approaches only used in novel situations or where problems occur, has a vision of what is possible

At each stage of development, there is progress in three different aspects of skilled performance. The learner moves from a reliance on abstract principles to using past concrete experiences as paradigms; from seeing the situation as a set of equally important bits to seeing it as a complete whole (where only some parts are relevant); and from being an observer in the situation to being thoroughly engaged.

Students benefit from sustained working alongside qualified practitioners. Ebright *et al.* (2004), who studied novice 'near miss' and adverse events, concluded that support for novice nurses in acute care environments should include consistent and available expertise. Workloads can be very unpredictable and experts can recognize risk and intervene prior to errors occurring, and expectations of novices need to be managed, even up to a year post-registration.

Benner (1984) advocated that novices should work alongside experts but elaborated little on what methods should be used to optimize learning through practice. Rogoff (1990) suggests that mentors and clinical supervisors can help novices with difficult problems by structuring sub-goals from the problem, focusing their learning on manageable aspects such as a certain skill required. Lauder *et al.* (2003) stress the significance of developing a 'reservoir' of knowledge and experience of particular cases so that the novice nurse builds a 'cognitive library' of nursing information for practice. Cassidy (2009, p. 36) discussed how mentors can share intuitive knowledge when engaged in dialogue as part of the student mentor relationship, calling this 'artistic sensitivity'; being able to see the difference between 'knowing that' say high standards of cleanliness are important to 'knowing how' to provide appropriate care for a vulnerable patient whilst assessing their emotional state.

Over to you

Accompany someone you recognize as an 'expert' in clinical practice during a clinical episode or patient interaction. The 'expert' and you have different viewpoints on this care episode. Spend time discussing what they and you think happened. The content and learning from the clinical episode is more easily visualized as you are talking about the clinical care close to the event.

What did the other practitioner do differently compared with what you would have done in the management of the clinical episode or care delivery?

Over to you

Examine the assessment tool used within the local health care practitioner education programme. Is there anything about this programme which appears to be based on Benner's model or any of the other level descriptors discussed here? If not, how might you find out about the underpinning knowledge that informed the development of this assessment tool?

Saliency
Knowing what matters to the person, through picking up cues, and acting on this

Moral agency
Provides information to empower others' decision-making, promotes dignity and respect and works with integrity

Determining expertise can be difficult. A concept analysis of the term 'expertise' (Manley and McCormack, 1997) identified:

- the attributes of holistic practice knowledge, knowing the patient, saliency, moral agency and skilled know-how
- the enabling factors of reflective ability, organization of practice, interpersonal relationships, autonomy and authority, and recognition by others.

The Royal College of Nursing Expertise in Practice project (Manley *et al.*, 2005) found that expertise, supported by critical reflective abilities, allowed experts to deconstruct their professional knowledge and artistry, but that this could also bring increased frustration with workplace constraints. Nurses with expertise were able to offer knowledgeable individualized care, using intuition, caring and empathy. 'Experts' were able to adapt and alter standard procedures and to change practice, where necessary, to meet the needs of service and patients, and their commitment to sharing their expertise was recognized by peers (Manley *et al.*, 2005).

Health care professional

Patient: identifying expertise

Paul has such a calm, approachable way with him that you genuinely believe him when he says, 'Give me a phone if you have any worries'. I know he must be really busy, but when you speak to him he gives you his full attention. He has so much knowledge about my problem and is very skilled, and he understands what this disease means to me. He helps me to navigate all the different departments that are involved in my care, and everyone who he works with thinks really highly of him. He's very professional without being 'stand-offish'.

> **Skilled know-how**
> Willing to share knowledge and skills, and act as a catalyst for change. Is able to take ethically reasoned risks, mobilizing all available resources

Critical thinking is an essential component of professional accountability and quality nursing care. Critical thinkers exhibit confidence, contextual perspective, creativity, flexibility, inquisitiveness, intellectual integrity, intuition, open-mindedness, perseverance, and reflection (Scheffer and Rubenfeld, 2000). Staib (2003) found that reflection, creativity, contextual perspective, and open-mindedness were the most common critical-thinking 'habits of the mind' addressed within nursing programmes and that, despite widespread interest in and recognition of the importance of developing critical-thinking skills, it was difficult to achieve.

This can also be compared to the development of mentorship practice as it is vital that new mentors learn from their expert colleagues, Benner's stages can be applied to mentorship (Table 7.1).

Table 7.1	Application of Benner's concept of novice to expert to the mentorship role
Level	**Mentor**
Novice	Undertaking preparation for mentorship. Behaviour based on own limited experience
Advanced beginner	Has completed the course but only beginning to mentor students with frequent support of senior practitioner. Awareness of existing outcomes
Competent	Mentoring students regularly but still requires support, able to manage most situations but reactive rather than proactive. Starting to interpret learning outcomes consistently
Proficient	Supervising others mentoring students, able to apply practice to any new learning needs. Experience of mentoring many different students. Able to manage difficult situations appropriately
Expert	Supporting others in a range of mentorship activities. Easy familiarity of all aspects of practice learning. Reliable assessor. Wide knowledge of educational processes, much experience of mentorship from all aspects

Developing as a mentor can be achieved through the completion of a mentor portfolio, where the mentor maps their practice to that of the NMC Standard to Support Learning and Assessment in practice (2008) which we discussed in Chapter 3.

MAKING SOUND JUDGEMENTS

It can be difficult for practice assessors to ensure the reliable assessment of clinical skills, knowledge and attitudes. Validity is crucial, and, as Ramsden (1992) suggests, much assessment in higher education is flawed, owing to the widespread use of surface approaches where the student does not need to show an understanding of fundamental ideas. We need to ensure that mechanistic and reductionist approaches to assessment are avoided, so that the practice of nursing is not being reduced to a set of tasks or competencies to be performed (Nicol and Freeth, 1998).

Watson *et al.* (2002) remind us that even when the definition of competence has been agreed there are issues with the assessment of it. Taylor *et al.* (2010) state that issues identified by Duffy (2004) regarding the expressed concerns around the validity and reliability of assessment tools, confirm the need for consistent, rigorous, well-valued assessment, adding that both 'who' and 'how' this is achieved being contentious topics for debate. Gopee (2008) identifies a 'practicability' factor.

As assessing practice is a complex activity, the practice aspect of a course has often been separated from the academic achievement and awarded only a pass or fail grade, even though many professional bodies require practice to have equal value to theory. Phillips *et al.* (2000b) found that in some scenarios assessment was viewed as a necessary but irksome 'bolt-on' activity.

Stuart (2007) argues that the core of any assessment is the judgement of the assessor – any form of assessment involves activity and judgment on the part of the assessor. She says that research suggests that the mentor's own concepts and interpretations play a very active role when making judgments and final assessment decisions, adding that these concepts and interpretations are likely to be influenced by the assessor's own competence and standards of practice.

Walsh (2010) reminds us that validity and reliability are the cornerstones of fair and objective assessment, adding that mentors need to be aware of factors that can influence an assessment. To have validity, an assessment should test what it is designed to test: therefore, the ability to administer drugs safely could not be assessed by questioning or discussion alone; it would require observation of drug administration undertaken by the student. For assessment to have reliability, different assessors should give similar scores for the same demonstration of care delivery, and summative assessment should relate to consistent performance. So, in the example of drug administration, if one mentor deems the student safe and effective in their drug administration, this should also be the case if another mentor witnesses this student's drugs' management on the same occasion.

Achieving high reliability means very simply that the judgements made in assessment can be trusted: 'inter' being between assessors – given the same student, in the same context, but a different assessor, the same conclusion will be reached; 'intra' being that an assessor, when utilizing effective and pertinent strategies, will reach a consistent quality of judgement. Reliability can be broadly perceived as conducting fair and accurate assessments (Stuart 2007). Whether something is valid or not is concerned with if it measures what it intends to measure, reliability refers to whether anyone else at any other time would reach the same conclusion (Fordham, 2005). Eraut (1998) suggests that if the discussion of competence is to be valuable then people need to be clear about the meaning, policy, rationale and context of the problem. A competency based assessment could be seen as being valid as it measures the skills and attributes it aims to in practice (McMullan, 2005) and according to Fordham (2005) the expertise of the assessor will influence the reliability of the assessment.

Reflective activity

Think about two occasions, one when you felt you were unfairly assessed and one where you felt fairly assessed. In each case, what factors led you to this viewpoint? Did the incident where you felt you were unfairly assessed affect your future learning?

Although assessment criteria assist objectivity, there are common pitfalls in the assessment process, which place validity and reliability at risk. Students' learning during clinical placements is, to a large extent, affected by the perceptions of assessors and students. Assessment that is based on discrete assessed episodes, such as an aseptic technique procedure, creates high anxiety levels and has a negative 'backwash' effect (Alderson and Wall, 1993). This type of assessment requires only lower-level cognition, such as factual recall or reproduction of a skill.

McMullan *et al.* (2003) reasons that professional judgement is central to assessment and the reliability of assessment is affected by the perspective taken and the training received. Gopee (2008) argues that practitioners have an ethical responsibility to patients to ensure that they assess accurately.

Reflective activity

Accountability for assessment within your professional career.

There is likely to have been a time when you have expressed the thought that a person should never have qualified (his or her attitudes or skills are appalling). What reasons might explain how this professional practitioner was in a position to qualify? How could you in your professional role prevent this situation from occurring?

EVIDENCE BASE

Read: Gopee, N. (2008) Assessing student nurses' clinical skills: The ethical competence of mentors. *International Journal of Therapy and Rehabilitation*, **15**(9): 401–407.

If we were given a task to do but not time or resources to complete it we would say it was unfair, and the same stands for assessment (Stuart, 2007). Therefore sufficient resources should be made available in terms of time for the students to practise and demonstrate competence; accessibility to appropriate learning opportunities in which skills and abilities can be developed; and also adequate time spent working with assessors to enable assessment.

GIVING AWARDS IN PRACTICE

Whether the course is vocationally or higher-education based, Jarvis and Gibson (1997) describe five basic requisites for assessing students:

1 look
2 listen (to what students say)
3 listen (to what others say about the students)
4 discuss
5 decide.

Woodcock (2009) has adapted the work of Hand (2006) and discussed four methods which follow a similar pathway. First, the assessor observes the learner when working with him or her so that communication skills and attitudes can be assessed, Questioning knowledge can identify gaps and a failure in application. Studying the testimonies of staff can ensure objectivity and assess progress, and lastly undertaking reflective discussions can reveal how students apply knowledge, evaluate their own practice and transfer learning.

KEY POINTS

When assessing clinical performance:

● Identify skills to be assessed

● Know what you would expect from a student at different stages in their programme, and make sure that you assess in line with the criteria

● Structure your working with a student to allow you to observe skills and behaviour as often as possible

● Gather information from a range of sources, e.g. student, other colleagues, patients

● Offer timely and constructive feedback

● Get students to discuss their rationales for their care

We will commonly assess 'intuitively' and whilst this is not wrong it is important that we check ourselves periodically to avoid subjective assessment relating to whether or not we 'like' the student rather than how well the student performs. Objectivity is required and this is sustained through making the initial level of expectation concrete within our minds. Adopting a systematic and structured approach will enable mentors to make accurate decisions in regard to the student's progress and their overall achievement (Aston and Hallum, 2011).

Andre (2000) advocates graded assessment because it can clarify for students the minimal competency requirements and also describe and record meritorious practice.

A pass/fail criterion for practice can be easier to use, as all that is required is to discriminate between safe and unsafe practice. Grading and banding require assessors to use criteria to discriminate between varying levels of practice and to reward a high level of achievement (Quinn and Hughes, 2007).

Over to you

The error of leniency is concerned with giving people the benefit of the doubt or being 'too soft' whereas the error of severity is the opposite, being too harsh or picking up on minor errors. In a central tendency error middle grades are given regardless of the quality of the performance, 'playing it safe' (Walsh, 2010).

Why do you think mentors might display errors of this type?

The 'halo' effect occurs when the student is judged with regard to their favourable personal characteristics (Quinn and Hughes, 2007). The concept that a 'good nurse' is synonymous with a 'nice person' continues in the minds of some assessors. It can be difficult for an assessor to decide that a student nurse has not met the assessment criteria when many of the clinical team have commented on what a nice, friendly team member he or she is.

Reflective activity

Think about someone who you have assessed in the past. Did you like them? Whether the answer was yes or no did it affect how you assessed them?

We need to recognize our own personal biases and ensure that these do not influence our judgements. Norm referencing can occur even when clear criteria are available for assessment judgements. Practitioners who work regularly with students encounter a variety of students and comparison of those who are at the same stage of training is difficult to avoid. Acknowledging that this can happen is the first step in reducing a 'norm-referencing effect'. If a mentor has recently worked with a second-year student who they perceived as excellent, the next second-year student on this placement may have their assessment compromised unless the mentor ensures that they assess using the explicit criteria provided by the education institute (criterion referencing).

RECOGNIZING EXPECTATIONS

Mentors must ensure that the assessment is appropriate for the level of learner (Walsh, 2010). Practice needs to be assessed and given an award right from the start of the student's time in placement. Within all assessment the assessor needs to prepare by having a level of expectation in relation to good, poor and excellent practice. It is useful to look at this from two different perspectives. Firstly be clear about your expectations of the specific performance or competency of 'the thing' you are assessing. What is your base line, what would you expect from a registered practitioner? Then identify what you expect from the current stage/level of learner. This can be where the grading, taxonomy or assessment criteria plays a very helpful part (see Figure 7.2.)

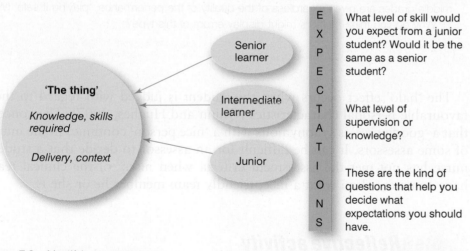

Figure 7.2   Identifying expectations

Developing assessment criteria that help assessors to discern the level of practice, and that are easy to use, can be a problem. Pfeil (2003) suggests that involving practitioners, mentors and lecturers in devising assessment criteria results in improved criteria for the summative assessment of practice.

Assessment criteria need to be easily related to learning outcomes. Evidence can be obtained through direct observation (e.g. watching the learner handle a dissatisfied patient), discussion (e.g. questioning and discussion about how a particular situation was/could be handled) and written information (e.g. reflective account in a learning journal, diary of a visit to Patient Advice and Liaison Service or the Complaints department). No single procedure is adequate for assessing clinical competence, so in the last example the more continuous the process of gaining evidence of achievement of the learning outcomes, the greater the predictive validity (Oliver and Endersby, 2000).

Biggs (2003) argues that criterion-referenced assessment, rather than norm-referenced, should be adopted and there should be a more holistic and divergent approach, involving significant peer and self-assessment. We looked at this briefly in Chapter 5, learners should be tested against assessment criteria rather than comparing to each other.

There are clear criteria for many of the tasks and care which we undertake set out within guidelines, Clinical Procedures and Trust Policies, e.g. Drug Administration, Patient Documentation, Discharge Planning, etc. Communication skills are often well known and understood in theory, yet in practice we continue to fail to apply this knowledge rigorously as there is no written policy or practice. Such skills may need to be made explicit by either the student or the assessor so that an acceptable 'standard' is agreed.

If it becomes necessary to remind a student of the required standard then the assessment may take on a formative nature, rather than summative (final) one. If the assessment has been arranged as a final/summative assessment then such a reminder **may** constitute a refer grade, where the prompting required has been over and above what you would expect for a student at that particular stage/level of their training. If most of the practice standard was recalled, or if the learner identified a gap in their knowledge and sought assistance in a timely manner, this may be a 'pass' in that the student has appropriately sought assistance and recognized their limitations. At this stage you can consider the detail of the awards. The stage of the course needs consideration, in relation to the complexity of the practice being assessed. At the end of year 1 it would not be unreasonable to award a pass for a student seeking assistance and clarification of practice, e.g. checking about follow up after abnormal vital signs but recognizing and reporting such abnormality safely. At the beginning of the final year the same student may not unreasonably be failed as such standards should be reaching a level of unconscious knowing – being second nature, e.g. noticing a subtle change in a patient's condition and checking vital signs independently. The grading of practice is complex yet it ensures that we, in turn, assess the complexity of clinical practice.

Student health care professionals may have learning difficulties that can affect their assessment. Mentors and assessors usually have limited knowledge of how to assist students who have dyslexia, for instance, and if not recognized this can lead to considerable assessment problems. Although this book can only offer limited guidance regarding this, perhaps the most important advice for students and mentors is that a confidential discussion early on in the placement can reduce the potential for problems within the assessment period. Mentors have a duty to ensure equality of opportunity for students with disabilities (Sharples, 2008).

TOP TIPS

When helping students who have told you that they have dyslexia:

- Provide pre-placement information, using Arial fonts (as these are easier to read).
- Ask them what their main difficulties are, and how you can help them.
- Ask questions clearly and concisely.
- Offer demonstrations and give clear instructions that are carefully sequenced.
- Allow practice in recording patient documentation, prior to requiring the student to contribute entries to patient records, and countersign all entries.
- Give time for student to independently calculate drug dosages, and always check these.

EVIDENCE BASE

Take a look at the following:

British Dyslexia Association **www.bdadyslexia.org.uk**
National Bureau for students with disabilities **www.skill.org.uk**

RCN (2010) *Dyslexia, dyspraxia and dyscalculia: a toolkit for nursing staff*, RCN: London.

TEACHING AND ASSESSING A SKILL

Teaching is a central aspect of mentorship, having the skill to recognize which approach or method to utilize is key, alongside an appreciation of learning theories and styles that we discussed in Chapter 5. We will generally explore teaching in the practice context further in the online bonus feature for this chapter. Being unable to perform procedures competently is stressful for a novice practitioner, so students are keen to develop skills. Skills can range from carrying out practical tasks (e.g. assisting with hygiene needs), to assessing patients (e.g. taking observations and interpreting these), to communicating (e.g. breaking bad news). Clinical skill laboratories, objective structured clinical examinations (OSCE) and manikins are increasingly being used to allow students to learn and assess skills in a safe environment, as it is not always practicable or ethical for some skills to be learnt initially in a clinical setting. However, such methods can only assist to a limited extent and students need to try out new skills with patients in clinical settings.

There are three main stages to teaching a skill:

1 Sensitizing students to the skill.
   They should be able to:

   - understand why the skill is important to them, both in the context of the course and in professional practice
   - analyze the skill in terms of its constituent parts
   - distinguish good practice from poor
   - evaluate the effectiveness of the skill when demonstrated.

2 Facilitating practice in the skill.
3 Giving feedback on the performance of the skill.
   Skills have been 'broken down' by Fisher *et al.* (2005) to incorporate reflections on skill development:

   - a definition/explanation of what it is you are trying to do (what is it?)
   - a rationale for the skill you are performing (why do it?)
   - what you need to know in order to do it (knowledge underpinning practice)
   - how to do it
   - sources of information (reference list)
   - reflection on how you did.

In the past, skills development was sometimes described as 'see one, do one and then teach one', but a preferred approach involves the supervisor breaking the demonstration of skills process into manageable steps. These steps can be:

1 **Demonstration** – the supervisor demonstrates skills at normal speed without any commentary.
2 **Deconstruction** – the supervisor demonstrates with an accompanying commentary.
3 **Comprehension** – the supervisor demonstrates with an accompanying commentary from the learner.
4 **Performance** – the learner demonstrates giving an accompanying commentary (Peyton, 1998).

Teaching a skill is linked to a judgement as to whether the learner can perform the skill adequately and a discussion about how the skill may be altered by differing circumstances. Using this approach to skill development encourages the student to move from 'consciously incompetent' to 'consciously competent', as shown in the 'Learning a skill' matrix in Figure 7.3 (Howell and Fleishman, 1982). Practice is the single most effective way to move from stages 3 to 4 in the matrix. The assessor can assess competence (can the student undertake this skill safely in a supervised environment?) and performance (are they able to practise this alone safely?).

Awareness

1. Unconsciously incompetent • the person is not aware that they have a particular deficiency in the area concerned • the person is not aware of the existence or relevance of the skill area	**2. Consciously incompetent** • the person is aware of their deficiency in this area, ideally through attempting or trying to use the skill • the person has a measure of the extent of their deficiency in the relevant skill, and a measure of what level of skill is required for their own competence
4. Unconsciously competent • the skill is so practised that it becomes 'second nature' • might now be able to teach others the skill concerned	**3. Consciously competent** • the person can perform the skill reliably at will • the person needs to concentrate and think in order to perform the skill

Practice

Figure 7.3   Learning a skill matrix, (reflects the thinking of Howell and Fleishman, 1982)

Steinaker and Bell (1979) developed an experiential learning taxonomy that is often used, sometimes in an adapted form, to assess the level of practice learning and skills achieved by a learner. This consists of:

1 **Exposure** – the student has observed the skill being performed by a competent practitioner.

2 **Participation** – the student has assisted a competent practitioner in the performance of the skill.

3 **Identification** – the student has performed the skill under the supervision of a registered practitioner.

4 **Internalization** – the student has sustained a skilled performance in a variety of settings under the supervision of a registered practitioner.

5 **Dissemination** – the student has maintained professional competence and has enabled others to develop their knowledge and skills.

An example of how this might be used in assessing the ability to administer drugs is given here.

Assessing the level of experiential learning (after Steinaker and Bell, 1979)

1   Exposure – the learner is introduced to the experience and is conscious of it as an observer. They should be able to describe some of the underpinning knowledge. (The implication is that the learner is not safe to participate as yet, even with supervision.) 'I watch another giving a patient their drugs.'

2 Participation – the learner has made a decision to become part of the experience, and participates under direct observation. (They may need prompting and guidance, and have a basic understanding of underpinning knowledge.)

'I administer drugs under close supervision.'

3 Identification – the learner identifies with the experience both intellectually and emotionally an Id is able to undertake care under supervision, but may require some guidance. (Is usually confident, safe and effective and able to discuss the application of knowledge.)

'I can competently administer drugs, although I still require them to be checked.'

4 Internalization – the learner's experience affects their behaviours and the way they do things, and they have the capacity to perform their practice with minimal guidance. (Is competent, safe and effective, and is able to demonstrate applied and situated knowledge.)

'Administering drugs is something I do most days when working clinically.'

5 Dissemination – the learner is now able to confidently execute skilled practice, to express the experience and advocate for others. They can also influence and teach others.

'I am skilful in drug administration and supervise and teach this to other staff and students.'

The criteria for assessment of performance should be clearly stated and specific, and high standards should be encouraged but these do need to be attainable. Students and assessors are often asked to assess the achievement of specified learning outcomes. The term 'learning outcome' encompasses what it is that a learner can do, what they understand, and what personal qualities and attributes they have as a result of their learning.

Assessment criteria for a competency can be specified using three domains of learning:

● the cognitive domain – knowledge outcomes concerned with the acquisition of knowledge (how we acquire information and what we need to know)

● the psychomotor domain – performance outcomes (relating to the development of skills and 'doing')

● the affective domain – attitudes and values displayed (formation of beliefs, values and attitudes).

Example of a learning outcome

By the end of the placement, the learner will be able to care for patients and relatives at times when they appear dissatisfied with an aspect of their care.

Knowledge outcomes

- Discuss the stages of dealing with patient and relative dissatisfaction from an informal response to a formal complaint.
- Describe the policies, guidance and role of the Patient Advice and Liaison Service (PALS) and Complaints Service.
- Discuss evidence available regarding patient satisfaction and dissatisfaction.

Performance outcomes

- Support and communicate effectively with patients and relatives who are dissatisfied with an aspect of care.
- Refer to PALS and Complaints colleagues where appropriate.
- Identify ways of improving satisfaction with patient care, informed by patient feedback.

Attitude and values

- Be empathetic and show respect towards patients and relatives who are dissatisfied with care.
- Appreciate good patient feedback, and recognize poor patient communication.
- Take a balanced and professional approach to all those involved in a complaints procedure.

Assessment criteria might be:

- The learner uses a polite and confident approach in all communications.
- The learner is able to decide rapidly whether they can manage the area of dissatisfaction with care in an appropriate manner, or whether they need to refer to a qualified practitioner.
- The learner is able to identify the route by which patients can access staff who can give advice on initiating a formal complaint.
- The learner is able to use evidence to inform changes to improve patient satisfaction with care.

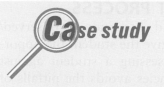

Case study

Assessing practice using grading criteria

Karen, an experienced mentor, is supervising three student nurses on clinical placement. When asked to outline the key features of their current level of practice to the link lecturer she describes them in the following way:

1 Grace is coming to the end of year one of her nurse training. She is a mature student who had a number of years' experience as a health care assistant prior to starting her nursing studies. She has good levels of practical skills and is hard working and able to use her initiative beyond that of many nurses at this stage of their course. Karen has noticed that Grace can be rather abrupt with patients who are quite dependent and sometimes seems to be concentrating on the task whilst excluding other aspects of care, such as her communication and her nurse–patient relationship development. When Karen asks Grace to discuss the underpinning rationale for her care, Grace says, 'I did it because I was asked to.'

2 Jack is an adult branch student of nursing at the end of his second year of studies. He appears to be rather hesitant in his delivery of care, and comes over as shy and nervous. He talks about his motivation to learn, but rarely uses his initiative and requires a lot of direction from Karen about what he is expected to achieve whilst on this placement. He is reliable in his work and has sound basic care skills. When questioned about what knowledge underpins his practice, Jack shows a sound understanding of the rationales for care.

3 Meena is near to the end of her third year of nurse training. She is a bright and energetic student, although sometimes she is a little immature in her discussions with colleagues and she has been reticent in identifying her personal learning needs. Meena has developed high-level clinical skills, shows motivation to learn and is sensitive to patient needs. She has needed considerable encouragement to display leadership skills, needing much prompting to undertake patient handovers, and gives succinct but insufficiently detailed reports of her observations.

Using the grading criteria for assessment of practice available in your locality, how do you think Karen would assess these three students' level of practice?

Looking at her accounts of the students, can you spot any potential risks in Karen's undertaking criterion-referenced assessment using these grading criteria?

Jasper and Fulton (2005) suggest that while portfolios have been used for some years in health care to assess professional attainment, the assessment process and criteria have mainly been rudimentary and underdeveloped. The criteria on which assessment is based are often locally developed, open to varying interpretations and adapted from existing higher education criteria, which are academically based, such as the Quality Assurance Agency for Higher Education's generic outcomes expected at different levels of academic study (QAAHE, 2001).

ISSUES AFFECTING THE ASSESSMENT PROCESS

Giving an award will often demand reflection and discussion of observed/demonstrated practice to clarify assumptions and give the student the opportunity to voice rationale and related theory. Assessing a student against predetermined criteria such as the NMC proficiencies avoids the pitfalls of subjectivity (Walsh, 2010). This type of technique is open to bias, the focus can veer away from the outcomes and instead be led by comparisons of students (Walsh 2010). Watson *et al.* (2002) ask what level of performance indicates competence. This is an area in which mentors can struggle, the use of assessment criteria being patchy and often open to interpretation (Finnerty *et al.*, 2006; Hyatt *et al.*, 2008).

There are growing recommendations to put in place ways of monitoring and auditing assessment (Wallace, 2003; Fordham, 2005; Hyatt *et al.*, 2008). This would enable the planning of development activity to inform preparation for mentorship programmes, recognition of good practice and the management of areas for improvement e.g., inter and intra mentor consistency. Quick reference guides in relation to assessment criteria could be developed and utilized (Hyatt *et al.*, 2008). See Figure 7.4.

Are you focused on assessment?

Feedback – Have you sought feedback from colleagues and service users?

Observation – Have you directly observed the student?

Criteria – Have you used the assessment criteria set out within the Assessment Documentation?

Understanding – Have you questioned your student's understanding and knowledge?

Scrutiny – Have you used documentation and evidence to assist you in your decision making?

Figure 7.4   A quick reference guide, (adapted from Gover and Heathershaw (2011))

This acronym was developed and produced on a small card as an aide memoire to assist any mentor in the assessment of their learner. It can be applied to any profession

EVIDENCING ACHIEVEMENT IN PRACTICE

Continuous assessment of practice often means that a portfolio of practice evidence is gathered to show achievement of the learning outcomes. A portfolio can be simply a tangible record of what someone has done, or a purposeful collection of materials that communicates a practitioner's development. McMullan *et al.* (2003) conducted a comprehensive literature review on the use of portfolios to assess holistic competence (including knowledge, skills, attitudes, performances and levels of sufficiency). A holistic way of viewing competence in portfolio assessment can help to overcome criticisms that assessment of competence can be fragmented, ignores context, lacks objectivity, and fails to assess knowledge, skills and attitudes in a comprehensive manner.

Scholes *et al.* (2004) looked at how mentors and nursing students match learning outcomes and competencies to their practice and then reconstruct experiences into the format required for the documentation within a portfolio. Portfolios enable assessors to measure student learning, help encourage reflective thinking, critical analytical skills, self-directed learning and provide detailed evidence of a practitioner's competence. To achieve maximum benefit from the portfolio there has to be a fit between the portfolio framework and the professional practice that is to be assessed (Scholes *et al.*, 2004). By engaging in a mentored, co-operative, and reflective process of portfolio development, students are able formatively to develop their self-assessment skills, make sense of what they were doing and plan their continuous improvement.

Endacott *et al.* (2004) identified four main forms of portfolio:

1 The shopping trolley – evidence is placed into a file with little structure and may include photocopies of articles and teaching notes, and resembles a resource file.

2 The toast rack – evidence is organized and slotted in under learning outcomes, but there is a large collection of papers, again including photocopied articles.

3 The spinal column model – uses competencies or learning outcomes to structure the portfolio, with the evidence being inserted behind each learning outcome and combined with a reflective commentary.

4 The cake mix model – this is a reflective commentary that asks the learner to show how and what they have achieved and learnt and how the evidence supports this.

Model 3 (spinal column) and Model 4 (cake mix) are most appropriate for health care professional education. Jasper and Fulton (2005) suggest that a general rule should be that the only evidence included should be referenced within a reflective review or a case should be made with regard to the learning outcomes. We also agree with Jasper and Fulton (2005) when they say that quality is more important than quantity in portfolio evidence.

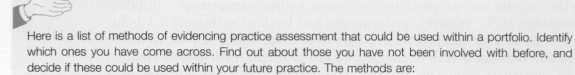

Over to you

Here is a list of methods of evidencing practice assessment that could be used within a portfolio. Identify which ones you have come across. Find out about those you have not been involved with before, and decide if these could be used within your future practice. The methods are:

- observation of practical skills
- student self assessment
- discussion
- learning contracts
- guided study
- written reflection
- testimony of others
- interviews
- patient comments and feedback
- peer evaluation
- audit or data collection
- case study
- team project.

Observation of practice

The mentor who is observing a learner is also an active participant in the clinical setting. It is easy for both the mentor and the learner to get carried away with delivering patient care in a clinical context, so much so that sometimes both can forget to record assessment evidence until a great deal later, which might reduce the richness and accuracy of the feedback. Observation is a powerful way to assess the practice of learners, giving an opportunity to observe learners at work and to compare this with what they say about their practice. It can be particularly motivating for a student to receive overt praise for exceptional practice, and the praise can be reinforced through written assessment records or testimonial statements. As the mentor observes, they progressively focus their attention on any issues that have started to emerge. Just watching and working alongside a student can be enough on which to base an assessment decision; however, it can be useful to triangulate this evidence by assessing understanding through discussion with the learner.

Over to you

Choosing and using evidence in a portfolio: think of a piece of evidence you have within your portfolio. Ask yourself the following questions about this piece of evidence.

1 What experience and knowledge do I already have and can demonstrate from this piece of evidence?

2 What are the implications professionally?

3 What practical examples can I give to demonstrate my skills and competence to support this evidence?

4 What other sources of evidence can I draw on to inform this section of my portfolio?

5 What literature could support this evidence?

6 How can I demonstrate best practice from this piece of evidence?

7 What ongoing/further development could I identify from this?

Not all the questions will be appropriate for each piece, but asking these makes you consider the reasons why you are including it and what other complementary evidence should be added.

When included within portfolios, discussions and the narrative accounts of practice allow assessors to examine specific and individual learning, rather than a more general, abstract discussion of practice.

EVIDENCE BASE

Obtain the following article and read the account of using reflective learning journals.
  Thorpe, K. (2004) Reflective learning journals: from concept to practice. *Reflective Practice*, **5**(3): 1–18.

Keeping a learning journal to inform reflective writing and narratives necessitates taking 'time out' from a busy day or dedicating time at the end of the day, but does allow the writer to figure out their learning. A learning journal is a record, enabling the learner to review, analyze, inform decision-making and action plan. Students are responsible for keeping their assessment of practice documentation during their placement, but should make this available whenever required by the mentor. One way of reviewing reflective learning accounts is offered here to assist those developing reflective evidence, as well as those who are responsible for assessment.

As suggested by Goodman (1989), another way of reviewing reflections on practice is to determine the level of the reflection using the factors outlined in Table 7.2.

Table 7.2 Assessing levels of reflection	
Level 1	Reflection to reach given objectives: Criteria are limited to issues of efficiency, effectiveness and accountability.
Level 2	Reflection on the relationship between principles and practice. There is an assessment of the implications, consequences and rationale for actions and beliefs.
Level 3	Reflection incorporates all of the above and in addition ethical and political concerns. Deliberations over the value of professional practice are included and the practitioner makes links between the practice setting and broader social structures.

(adapted from Goodman, 1989)

Assessment indicators for reflective work (adapted from Moon, 1999)

Purpose

● The student should demonstrate understanding of the purpose, selection and description of the issues on which they reflect.

Description of an event or issue

● Description is present and provides an adequate focus for reflection.
● Description includes statement of observations, comments on personal behaviour, comments on reactions/feelings, comments on context.

Additional information

● Relevant knowledge, theory, experience and feelings
● Suggestions from others
● New information
● Other factors, e.g. ethical, moral, political and contextual

Reflective thinking

● Able to structure the material – was an identified reflective framework used?
● Was theory linked to practice?
● Was the viewing of issues/events from different points of view?
● Evidence of new ideas being tested in practice or revisited and revised.

A conclusion

● A statement of either what has been learnt, solved or actions that relate to the incident or area of practice.
● Identification of a new area for further reflection.

A difficult aspect of working in health care is acknowledging your own beliefs and values and recognizing that they may be very different from the beliefs and values held by your clients or patients and your peers. Reflective writing within a portfolio allows you to explore your professional values and beliefs. However, Orland-Barak and Wilhelem (2005) found that some nursing students used procedural professional language in their accounts of their learning, concentrating their narratives on describing biomedical care procedures, such as changing a colostomy bag, with rarely any deeper-level reflection being offered. This focus is understandable from a 'novice' perspective where skill performance is often a priority. Orland-Barak and Wilhelem (2005) take the view that it is important to allow student nurses time to look at the instrumental aspects of practice, as this is a novice's starting point for making sense of practice. Novices have been characterized as concrete in their thinking, using this form of reasoning because initially they need to adopt a single perspective on a problem before they can learn sensitivity to varying contexts. Mentors should allow students time to work on these fragmented aspects of practice, whilst encouraging them to transform these procedural and instrumental ways of thinking about practice into integrated personal and professional reflections.

ACCREDITATION OF PRIOR LEARNING

Workplace learning has become increasingly valued, for instance the accreditation of prior experiential learning (APEL). The fundamental principle of accreditation of prior (experiential) learning is that learning through experience is capable of gaining recognition and credit, regardless of the time, place and context where it is achieved, and is not dependent on any formal setting.

- Accreditation of prior learning can be matched to the learning outcomes that can be gained through formal qualification, with learners seeking 'credit' for showing how their experiential learning matches that of the qualification.
- The outcomes from prior certificated learning can be matched to outcomes of a formal qualification in order to gain exemption from particular modules.
- Accreditation of prior learning can be used as an alternative entry qualification to join a programme (termed 'advanced standing').

It is rare, however, for an entire qualification to be formed through the basis of past achievements alone. Evidence used in assessing prior learning may be direct (e.g. reflective writing, teaching plans, assignments, projects, articles) or indirect (e.g. certificates or witness testimonies).

Macdonald and Savin-Baden (2004) advocate that assessment of learners should ideally:

- be based in a practice context in which students will find themselves working in the future

- assess what the professional does in their practice, which is largely process-based professional activity, underpinned by appropriate knowledge, skills and attitudes
- reflect the learner's development from a novice to an expert
- encourage learners to appreciate and experience the fact that in a professional capacity they will encounter patients, clients, users, professional bodies and peers, who will continue to 'assess' them
- engage learners in self-assessment and reflection as the basis for future continuing professional development and self-directed learning
- consider the extent to which assessment practices are inclusive or whether they discriminate against certain students.

This chapter has provided you with an overview of assessment and the forms of evidence that can be used within portfolios. The movement from novice to expert practice has also been explored.

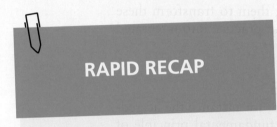

RAPID RECAP

Check your progress so far by working through each of the following questions.

1 What are the key differences between:

   (a) formative and summative assessment of practice

   (b) criterion-referenced and norm-referenced assessment of practice?

2 What are the level identifiers within Steinaker and Bell's (1979) experiential taxonomy?

3 Identify at least six forms of evidence that could be included within a practice portfolio.

4 What methods can you use to assess practice?

5 What should be done about patient information, when placing evidence that links to patient care practice into an assessment-of-practice document?

If you have difficulty with one of these questions, read through the section again to refresh your understanding before moving on.

CHAPTER 8

TECHNOLOGY IN 21st CENTURY PRACTICE, LEARNING AND TEACHING

LEARNING OBJECTIVES

By the end of this chapter you should be able to:

- explain how using technology in education can enhance learning

- identify a range of technologies which are available

- appreciate the importance of remaining focused on the learning outcome

- start to identify opportunities for using technology in practice learning

Bonus features for this chapter available on the book's website

INTRODUCTION

In this chapter we will explore some of the technology used to enhance, support and complement practice learning. It is also useful to appreciate the learning experience of students when they are studying the theoretical aspects of their programme. Some of you may be students yourselves as part of your continuing professional development or you may be required to access 'e-learning' as part of your mandatory training. Whatever your position your skill and knowledge in this area is likely to be variable.

The intention of this chapter is to give you an overview and flavour of the current technological innovations and considers the impact on us as mentors and educators. A caution though as we are all aware the pace of change is enormous so even when we feel we have grasped a particular strategy it may already have moved on!

BACKGROUND

The use of the Internet and the World Wide Web has increased exponentially beyond comprehension. In our everyday lives and practice we encounter technology all the time, maybe even taking it for granted. Even if we do not use this at home directly we perhaps communicate electronically at work via email or buy our groceries in a supermarket where we can scan the goods ourselves. Foret Giddens *et al.* (2010, p. 355) say that we are 'in the midst of a technological revolution which touches all aspect of our lives' adding that it's use in education is an expectation. Selwyn (2011) concurs with this, feeling that the use of technology in education has become so widespread that it appears to be viewed as common sense.

Educationalists are responsible for developing the learning material, teaching content and session outcomes. As with other forms of delivery an appreciation of learning theories and styles is necessary (see Chapter 5). Strategies to deliver these will be developed. At its most basic level the way that technology is utilized to communicate with each other in education has increased the consistency and quality of information that is shared. Students have a different experience to that of their forbears, this is a natural progression, but essentially they are learning to become the same practitioner albeit one fit for the 21st century. An experienced colleague gave some advice to a fellow lecturer when they began to encounter technology in education, he said: remember your learning outcomes do not change because you are using technology, the only thing that has changed is that you won't physically be face to face with your students, you need to decide how to meet the outcomes in a different way. Naturally this does have an effect on the contact between the student and teacher however, not being able to 'see' your students in a face to face environment necessitates interacting in a different way.

Being able to develop teaching and learning materials provides a rich opportunity to draw on a variety of sources which suit the needs of a range of learners. Edwards (2012) suggests that many herald the increased use of computers in education as the new age, with many benefits, including that of accessibility, meeting the needs of a variety of learners. However Selwyn (2011) says that in the same way that people are concerned with energy consumption but use fridges, we should be giving attention to the activities and meanings that are attached to the technological devices, tools and applications in education, not just the devices, tools and applications themselves.

Student

Health student

When I started my course one of the first things that we were introduced to was the university's intranet and programme area, the way that we communicate with our lecturers and the course administration team as well as being able to access material about the our learning modules and the actual course itself. I can email my personal tutor or course leader, read announcements about my course as well as the social side of being a student even when I'm out in practice. I still feel like a member of the university even when I'm not there.

Technology can be understood simply as the process by which humans modify nature to meet their needs and wants (Selwyn, 2011, p. 7) 'doing things better'; inclusive of what technologies actually are, how they are used and the social structures surrounding them. Some individuals see technology as something tangible, for example a piece of machinery, however it could be argued that knowledge is also involved in this in as much as understanding and skill may be required to use this piece of machinery in the correct way (Edwards, 2012).

It seems that very quickly terms such as 'wikis', 'blogs' and so on are being used in a learning capacity; recognizing what these are and how they can be utilized in collaborative learning can be intimidating to the uninitiated. There are many examples available to draw on: augmented reality simulators to gain proficiency in suturing skills (Botden *et al.*, 2009); wikis that can be used to create a shared document (Collier, 2010); podcasts to record supplementary content (Lymn and Bowskill, 2010); video mediated technologies for one to one support (Taylor and Nichol, 2011); the use of serious games in the acquisition of community health nursing skills (Hogan *et al.*, (2011); next generation learning spaces (Wilson and Randall, 2012) to mention only a few.

Remaining focused on the intended learning outcome is key however, not simply to use technology because it is fashionable or available. Social scientists would suggest that technology is value laden and linked to cultural and environmental influences (Edwards, 2012). This means that when developing and using resources, attention should be paid to the impact of this facility. What could the subsequent impact be? Is accessibility equitable between student groups? Is the effect the same in a different context, for example, in rural areas? Including material which enables the learner to access a wealth of resources potentially from around the world, can only supplement and compliment those already in existence.

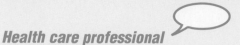

Health care professional

Nurse lecturer

I tell my students at the start of their course, don't be scared of technology. It is there to aid learning and teaching. Remember it can enhance your experience. Just as you once worried about sending a text or mobile banking it becomes part of the whole experience. Don't frame learning as 'chalk and talk' from previous experiences. Technology is one of the many ways of enriching what we learn and experience in the virtual or real class room setting.

KEY POINTS

- The use of the World Wide Web and technology has increased beyond comprehension

- The use of technology in education has become widespread.

- The learning outcome should be the focal point when developing approaches to teaching and learning activities.

MODELS AND APPLICATIONS

The use of technology as with other disciplines has philosophical perspectives, it is not within the remit of this chapter to explore these in depth but an awareness of these can assist with understanding how experts may approach the subject.

One view point is that of 'technological determinism', this is based on the premise that technology is an independent self-regulating phenomenon which shapes the future itself rather than as a result of human aspirations and desires (Edwards, 2012), an element of inevitability being involved. So in the way that the human race and the world have progressed technology has also.

There is also a constructivist viewpoint that maintains that by reflecting on our own experiences we create our own understanding of the world (Edwards, 2012). This evolved into the model of social construction of technology in part as a response to the pessimistic viewpoint of inevitability. This proposes that there is a link between social and technical processes and suggests that they are both human constructs. Technology evolves through an organic or evolutionary process (Edwards, 2012).

These are complex concepts to grasp, however they can offer an interesting perspective to reflect on when we look at how we utilize technology in curriculum development activities, for example. Fundamentally according to Edwards (2012) technology in education is difficult to grapple with, it has advanced over time and could equally include things such as devices, as well as systems and processes. He sees that this presents us with a unique challenge, whether technology is neutral or as highlighted before, involving values.

Magnussen (2008) suggests that e-learning technologies draw on adult learning theories that view the educator as a facilitator. This fits with our experience, the learner can have much more freedom to engage and influence the direction and pace of their learning. As a clinical educator or practitioner you will no doubt have already engaged with technology from a clinical perspective in the way that you provide your service or deliver practice and in a similar vein source material as part of your own continuous professional development as well as supporting learners and contributing to the richness of the clinical learning environment.

Reflective activity

Reflect on how you use technology in your practice.

How has this changed in the last few years? What equipment do you use in your everyday practice? How is client care recorded?

THE VIRTUAL LEARNING ENVIRONMENT

With the advent of the Internet and World Wide Web, educationalists have begun to realize that much activity in this virtual world has significant implications for learning and teaching and is often communal in nature (Edwards, 2012). Learners, mentors and academia have the opportunity to communicate and interact with each other in contemporary ways. The virtual learning environment as we know it is a 'learning platform' that is used as a repository for information, teaching and learning materials, submission of work for assessment and vehicle for giving feedback. Teaching and learning materials may include links to articles, podcasts, interactive quizzes, videos, links to webpages and so forth.

According to Edwards (2012) the increasing use of technology has resulted in bringing the discussion of whether communication between learners and teachers should be synchronous or asynchronous to the forefront. Synchronous communication occurs simultaneously and requires participants to engage in real time but not necessarily in the same place whereas asynchronous communication is also free of the need to be in the same place but is not dependent on simultaneous exchanges (Edwards, 2012). The latter can be quite revelatory as free of time and space.

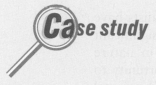

Over to you

Look at these two examples. What do you think might be the benefits of each approach? What might the challenges be?

Synchronous communication

Software was utilized to hold a 'virtual' lesson. All learners agreed a particular time for the session and accessed this on the Web via a login link which had been emailed to them. The facilitator was able to share their own computer screen on which a presentation was given in real-time. The students, by use of headphones and microphones, were able to talk to each other and ask questions of the facilitator. All participants were at home.

Asynchronous communication

Learners were asked to reflect on a change in practice that they had been involved in. They were then invited to share their experiences with their fellow students via an online blog.

The decision on which method of communication to use should be based on learning needs rather than other factors (Edwards, 2012). Both could be employed, this would give rise to a blended approach. Using a variety of approaches for teaching and learning is not a new concept in itself of course (Edwards, 2012), for many years teachers have considered using a variety of strategies. Employing a blended approach to learning can provide a unique and rich environment for learning, however the development of useful material in my experience requires a significant amount of preparation time, partly due to the changed relationship and interaction between the teacher and learner, particularly if an asynchronous approach is used.

Case study

A mentor preparation team were reviewing the content and delivery of their programme. Student evaluation remained positive, however the volume of content necessitated very full sessions with decreasing time for discussion. Individuals on the team were very passionate about the impact and importance of mentorship but wanted to utilize this review as an opportunity to enhance the student's learning experience and reinvigorate the programme.

The previous structure consisted of six days with face to face sessions and a significant amount of information provided in module area of a 'useful resource/ further reading/ simple links' variety. The proposed structure was to move to each day having a face to face taught element in the morning with a 'virtual' component in the afternoon, three of which would ask for work to be submitted.

The content was divided between the team and themes for each day were developed. A range of learning materials and activities were utilized. These included using video clips, completing interactive quizzes, signposting learners to case studies and reading material, and recording podcasts. This has resulted in the acquisition of new skills for the course team and an innovative experience for the learner.

What do you think that some of the challenges might be with introducing this type of blended learning approach?

Discussion Whilst the feedback from students has been positive some recurring comments have been received. These centred on securing enough time to become familiar with the technology, which could distract from the content. This was anticipated to a degree and so further support was offered. One element which was beyond the control of the course team was the functionality of individual learner's hardware; advice from technology support teams was sought as to utilizing most basic requirements in terms of operating systems and equipment. Some learners report being unable to access some material so alternative sources were provided.

Virtual worlds have a three dimensional capacity, they can be interactive and simulate space (Edwards, 2012), they can be occupied through the use of avatars and take on an experiential aspect in a potentially unlikely range of contexts that extend the notion of learning by doing. Attention should be given however to factors such as moral principles and ethics, educators need to understand how to use this technology effectively and bridge the divide between virtual gaming and learning (Edwards, 2012). By inventing themselves in the form of an avatar an individual may 'perfect' themselves, so the behaviour displayed or responses given are prospective and fall under the heading of 'should'.

There are a variety of virtual world applications which have been used, these include: Penfield Virtual hospital (Ward and Hartley, 2006), problem based learning spanning real and second life worlds (Good et al., 2008) Stilwell (Walsh and Crumbie, 2011) The Neighbourhood (Giddens et al. 2010) This type of innovation has gained the interest of nursing educators as it has the potential to frame nursing in a way that is realistic and relevant to all learners (Giddens et al., 2010). Giddens et al. expressed a concern however that such is the rapid rise of this, there is a need for evaluation in order to gain an understanding of what and how students learn from virtual communities. In the online bonus feature accompanying this chapter we will consider how an interactive resource can be designed.

E-PORTFOLIOS

As identified in Chapter 6 health care professionals are expected to maintain a professional portfolio, this can take an electronic form offering an innovative way to meet registration requirements (Moores and Parks, 2010). However, e-portfolios can be used for a variety of different purposes (Whitsed, 2005). They can be used for personal development, the presentation of work or for assessment activities.

Students can add to an e-portfolio as they travel through educational institutions (Whitsed, 2005), this transfers across into the tenet of lifelong learning where a practitioner could draw on previous learning to demonstrate perhaps application to work or skills development. There can be advantages for both the practitioner/learner and the educational institution: the opportunity to utilize a tool which from the learner's perspective gives new ways to record and present material which support employment, and as an HEI encourages and develops independent and reflective learners (Whitsed, 2005).

Following a trial of e-portfolios with occupational therapy and physiotherapy students, Moores and Parks (2010) developed 12 tips for introducing e-portfolios with undergraduate students (see Table 8.1).

Table 8.1 Twelve tips for implementing an e-portfolio	
Tip 1	**Identify the added value of using an e-portfolio** – it is not merely a computerized version, many more options offered.
Tip 2	**Consider the long and short term use of an e-portfolio** – it can be utilized for a specific module but also throughout an individual's career
Tip 3	**Consider when and how the e-portfolio is introduced** – timing needs to be carefully considered, not necessarily at induction
Tip 4	**Enable students to develop a personal learning space** – other methods are usually controlled by the HEI but in this instance the e-portfolio remains private to the student, they define who can see what.
Tip 5	**Use a function of an e-portfolio to submit an assessment to maximize motivation** – increase motivation to learn to use effectively
Tip 6	**Assessment guidelines should be transparent but not too prescriptive** – they should be written with the function of the e-portfolio in mind, traditional marking criteria such as word counts may not be appropriate
Tip 7	**Provide students with clear guidance on confidentiality and the use of digital media** – really important to provide guidance especially in regard to confidentiality, e.g. who should electronic information be shared with even if it is the tutor.
Tip 8	**e-portfolios do not teach reflective practice** – students will need to be guided to develop skills in reflection
Tip 9	**Use the e-portfolio to give feedback** – again motivation will be raised if given early and is constructive
Tip 10	**Ensure that students can access their e-portfolio** – availability of hardware is essential
Tip 11	**Make use of internal support available within the institution** – draw on technical support
Tip 12	**Do not reinvent the wheel** – although not commonplace many HEIs have used e-portfolios experiences and recommendations are easily available

(Adapted from Moores and Parks, 2010)

In our opinion these tips offer a balanced and very useful perspective if considering using an e-portfolio. If they are to be used for assessment purposes, e-portfolios can allow different media to be submitted which print versions do not, for example video and audio files, images (Whitsed, 2005). Students can also participate in their own assessment when using e-portfolios by identifying strengths and weaknesses as well as personal progress over time (Skiba, 2005). E-portfolios are often used on a longitudinal basis, as an all round activity. Referring to using an e-portfolio, when in fact the meaning is really only electronic submission of a workbook, which was previously submitted as a hard copy is not quite the same thing.

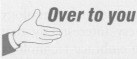

Over to you

Whitsed (2005) identified project work occurring in the UK – look at this website; there is some interesting information about the use of e-portfolios. http://www.eportfolios.ac.uk

Have you had any experience with using an e-portfolio?

MOBILE TECHNOLOGY AND LEARNING

Mobile learning provides the opportunity for anyone to access information and learning materials from anywhere and at anytime through the use of wireless technology (Ally, 2009). It is in this area that mentors, educators and practitioners may come into contact with technology when supporting their learner. This could be simply being aware that students can access the university virtual learning environment, communication systems for emails or complimentary learning resources such as online journals via the Web.

This facility allows for high level learning as individuals can access and apply information straight away rather than one after the other as in previous experiences (Ally, 2009). There is no need to 'wait' until later and look something up after a shift, for example.

According to Traxler (2009) the use of mobile technology is gradually increasing and diversifying across every sector of education. Most recently a colleague presented a poster at a conference; on this poster was an image: and by using augmented reality technology on a mobile phone application and scanning the image, conference participants were able to access a video when pointing their devices at the poster.

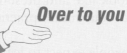

Over to you

Read this article – Traxler, J. (2010) Students and mobile devices. *ALT-J Research in Learning Technology,* **18**(2): 149–160. This is an online open access journal.

Have you had any experience of using mobile learning technologies? Can you think of a resource that you could use to enhance your practice?

THE FUTURE

Strachan *et al.* (2011) undertook a survey into the effectiveness of technology to support work-based learning, this demonstrated very interestingly that whilst students were positive there was a reluctance to embrace technology from some of the academic staff. The study concluded that all parties should be reminded to ensure that the quality of the delivery of the online programme should be paramount if it was to be fit for the 21st century. Skiba (2005) advises that there are critical elements which influence the successful implementation of e-portfolios: as a priority a culture of understanding and support should be created. This is an important point: to enhance the learning experience sufficient preparation and resource must be given to the creation of teaching and learning materials and the infrastructure that provides support.

Such is the pace of development in digital technology educational technologists manage to just keep abreast of their topic without the ability to study more complex issues that underpin these endeavours (Selwyn, 2011). One very interesting point made by Edwards (2012) is that one outcome of the technological advance is that those who have grown up with computers will exceed those who have not. Having said this even now technology is not just an endeavour of the young but it is embedded in compulsory education from the start.

Selwyn (2011) reminds us that predicting the future remains a risky business, nevertheless the need to assess accurately the potential impacts of technology on society and indeed education, is an essential part of attempting to control and manage technology. Buchan (2011) unearthed a 'chicken and egg' situation when examining the transformational impact of learning technology, whilst learning technology is an important part of the future, organizations need to have the foresight, capacity and adaptability to meet this challenge.

Educationalists should make decisions based on what the future might hold (Edwards, 2012). Factors such as affluence, the global economy, future working patterns, demographics and social cohesion will shape this. But of course we can only ponder on what the future might look like and presume that 'based on our knowledge, expertise and experience' our future practice may require certain skills to develop.

Some things are more certain though. The fact that people expect to learn, work and study wherever and whenever they want has been identified as a key trend in the next five years (Johnson *et al.*, 2012). The New Media Consortium Horizon Report 2012: Higher education edition (Johnson *et al.*, 2012) highlights emerging technologies with considerable potential, areas in which work is already taking place. On the horizon within the next 12 months are mobile apps and tablets; game-based learning and learning analytics will appear in the next two to three years and gesture-based computing and the 'Internet of things' in four to five.

Some of us are already using mobile apps with ease, games have always been used to learn and many of us have experienced using gesture based gaming in our own homes.

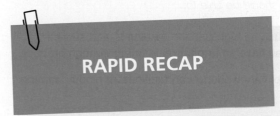

Over to you

Read this editorial

McGonigle, D. and Eggers, R. (2001) Editorial: Introduction – A student in the not too distant future. *Online Journals of Nursing Informatics (OJNI)* **15**(2) available at **http://ojni.org/issues/?p=620**

What do you think the possibilities might be?

In this chapter we have discussed how technology can and is being used in the education programmes which make up part of health care provision now. You will be familiar with some of this technology even if you haven't previously considered it consciously or applied it to the acquisition of knowledge or skills.

RAPID RECAP

Check your progress so far by working through each of the following questions.

1 What is the difference between synchronous and asynchronous communication?

2 List the key components of mobile learning

3 Explain how an e-portfolio can be used

4 Describe what a virtual learning environment is.

If you have difficulty with any of these questions, read through the section again to refresh your understanding before moving on.

FURTHER READING

JISC (2012) Crossing the Threshold: moving e-portfolios into the mainstream available from **http://www.jisc.ac.uk/publications/programmerelated/2012/crossingthethreshold.aspx**

JISC (2012) Learning in a digital age available from **http://www.jisc.ac.uk/publications/programmerelated/2012/learning-in-a-digital-age.aspx**

CHAPTER 9

INFLUENCES ON THE QUALITY OF PRACTICE LEARNING

LEARNING OBJECTIVES

By the end of this chapter you should be able to:

● understand how issues, such as high patient caseloads and service improvement initiatives, can have an impact on learning through practice

● appreciate how multidisciplinary working can facilitate or hinder learning through practice

● acknowledge the role of emotional labour within health care

● recognize effective strategies to minimize the effect of constraints within varying contexts of practice.

Bonus features for this chapter available on the book's website

INTRODUCTION

Everyday work in clinical settings has, understandably, patient care as the priority and this can be viewed as constraining learning through practice. Busy workloads and the emotional content of health care delivery can create stress, when combined with providing support for learners. This chapter explores possible barriers to work-based learning, such as high patient case-loads, professional agendas, emotional labour and variations within different clinical settings. Ways to manage these constraints to learning through practice are discussed. Personal barriers to an individual's learning through practice, such as diminished self-confidence, being defensive to feedback and being uncomfortable with self-evaluation, have been explored in Chapter 5, so are not discussed in any depth here. Many factors can hinder or facilitate learning; some of these factors are identified in Figure 9.1.

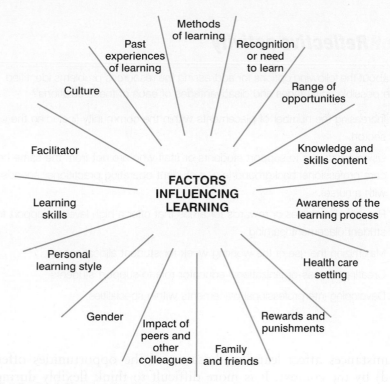

Figure 9.1   Factors influencing learning
(adapted from Connexions (2003) *Learning and Young People.* Department for Education and Skills, p. 12)

Emotional labour
The actions an individual undertakes to manage their feelings when there is a gap between what they actually feel, and what they think they should feel. The term emotional labour indicates the emotional work done as part of a job and is governed by 'feeling rules' set by the employer. These unarticulated rules of social interactions indicate how deeply we should feel and for how long. Expectations for emotional labour tend to be linked to female-dominated work roles

RESOURCE ISSUES

Staff shortages can hamper learning, as existing practitioners need to manage high workloads and there is an increased reliance on temporary staff. Employment changes to improve working lives include allowing and encouraging flexible working and making sure there is a suitable work–life balance, but increases difficulties for senior staff having to cover 24-hour care requirements and can make it difficult to roster students and their mentors together. With part-time working on the increase, a single student may work with a number of registered practitioners during their placement. Recruitment and retention is important as the loss of experienced staff affects the continuity of care and the overall learning environment in the clinical area. Also, shortages of placement opportunities in certain specialities can be compounded by the lack of adequately prepared clinical educators. Taking the time to meet with a clinical supervisor has benefits, however if staff are 'working flat out' this has a potentially detrimental effect on professional development.

Reflective activity

Think about the following options for addressing the resources problems identified. What are the possible advantages and disadvantages of each of these solutions?

- Increasing the number of placements within the community (including the private sector).
- Using educators to support students or staff who are not from the same health care professional background (e.g. a student operating practitioner spends time with a nurse).
- Providing incentives or rewards for areas that offer a high level of support for student placement learning.
- Maximizing the use of the working week for student allocations.
- Creating a cross-organizational educator role to support students.
- Developing interprofessional placements within specialities.

Circumstances affect learning, because of the opportunities offered (or withheld) by the context. It is more difficult to think flexibly during times of tension and stress so it is understandable that nurses and other health care professionals often act, think and behave in their 'usual' way even though this may not fit the situation (McAllister, 2003). Available evidence, the level of complexity and the practitioner's capabilities and disposition are factors that link with context to affect thinking. The time available and the complexity of the situation are important variables, and shortages of time force people to adopt a more intuitive approach, and intuitive routines help experienced staff to do things more quickly (Eraut, 2000b). Although routines vary between different clinical settings, the situated learning of these routines and the ability to perform accepted practice fluently within a setting is important to membership of a clinical team (Wigens, 2004).

Over to you

Here is an example of a morning routine within one medical ward:

07.00   Handover from night shift to both teams. All patients are to have their observations and other charts reviewed and updated.

07.20   Handover is completed and drugs round commenced. Assist some patients who wish to meet washing and hygiene requirements prior to breakfast. Prepare patients for breakfast.

08.00	Serve breakfasts, giving assistance to those who require it. Document any food diaries and fluid charts. Once protected food time is complete, continue to assist other patients with hygiene needs. Ensure care is documented. Intentional care round.
09.00	Day-specific commitments are commenced, e.g. preparation of patients for discharge, ward rounds.
10.00	Record any observations. Intentional care round.
10.30	Staff breaks commence.
11.45	All staff should have returned from break.
11.45	Record any blood sugar measurements required.
12.00	Any patients with confirmed discharges should have departed; the reasons for any delays should be documented. Prepare patients for lunch (protected mealtime). Intentional care round.

How useful do you think this ward routine would be to staff and students within this area? Find out about any routine within your current area of practice. Is this documented or simply in the heads of the staff in the area?

Professionals may be reluctant to talk about routines if they feel that these differ from those espoused in theories (such as individualized care) as they think that doing so will highlight inadequacies. Time pressure and uncertainty induce changes in the cognitive strategies used, influencing both the process and quality of decisions. Among the coping strategies utilized in situations of uncertainty are the use of planning schedules and the synchronization of tasks, and there can be value in having a certain level of routine, but this needs to be delivered in an ethos of meeting the individual needs of patients. One example of this is care or intentional rounding. A number of high-profile reports have drawn attention to examples of poor standards of fundamental nursing care – attending to patients' needs for support with feeding, positioning, personal hygiene and skin integrity (Parliamentary and Health Services Ombudsman, 2011).

At the same time, there is a growing body of evidence that suggests more nursing time per patient results in better patient outcomes (Dix *et al.*, 2012, Kings College London, 2012). This includes carrying out regular checks with individual patients at set intervals, typically hourly – two hourly when they are in-patients. During these checks nurses carry out scheduled or required tasks. Care rounding helps frontline teams to organize ward workload to ensure all patients receive attention on a regular basis. What is critical to this approach is reliability and consistency. The round begins with opening words, in which carers introduce themselves and explain why they are there to build patients' trust and confidence. The staff follow this up by carrying out scheduled tasks or observations with patients; addressing patients' pain, positioning and toilet needs; assessing and attending to the patient's comfort; and checking the environment for any risks to the patient's comfort or safety. The round also includes closing key words – typically: 'Is there anything else I can do for you – I have time, and will be back again when your next medication is due', and making sure that the call bell is in reach. Finally, rounds are documented, which fulfils audit requirements. These care rounds have been found to reduce call bell usage, increase patient satisfaction, reduce patient falls and also pressure ulcers.

Uncertainty can be defined as the variability, degree of complexity, or novelty of a particular situation, and is linked to the character of the information available. Those who feel in control of their environment perceive uncertainty as a challenge, rather than as a threat, and are more likely to respond to this, using problem-solving strategies (Schuler and Jackson, 1986).

There are a number of strategies for coping with time pressure and information overload, including speeding up (acceleration), selecting the input of information (filtering), prioritizing, using 'decision rules', omitting or avoiding, and locking on to one approach. When stress is high, a decision is likely to be made based on what has previously been successful, and this decision may not be based on knowledge of all the available alternatives.

Learning to cope with (or even override) stress is part of 'situated learning' (Wigens, 2004). Nurses learn to assess, sort, and reshuffle the prioritization of patients in their care. This prioritization often uses a guiding framework, such as focusing on the 'sickest' patients and putting off aspects of care (such as support and advice giving) until later. By reviewing what has been provided, and looking back on past experiences, this guiding framework is evaluated for trustworthiness. Being able to constantly prioritize at speed and handle uncertainty whilst appearing calm and in control of the situation is the sign of an experienced nurse and something to which new staff nurses aspire.

Reflective activity

Think about the prioritization frameworks used in your current area of work. Have they been made explicit? Could you outline them to a colleague?

Changes in skill mix that increase the level of non-registered staff may also affect learning through practice. Skill mix involves professionals being willing to accept a form of interprofessional working that recognizes the possibility that some needs may be met more effectively by lesser-trained staff. Skill mix can be achieved through delegation, substitution or diversification. However, there can be ambivalence within a nursing team about the role of support staff. Nurses value the contribution of assistants, but whether nurses accept this group as part of the nursing family is still open to debate (RCN, 2003).

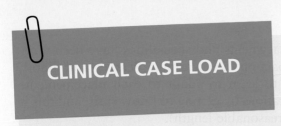

CLINICAL CASE LOAD

Therapists need to delegate care delivery to assistants safely and in line with training. Saunders (1998) suggests a framework of questions (originally developed for physiotherapists). If the answers to the questions are yes, the delegation should be safe, but it remains the responsibility of the qualified nurse to provide supervision for the health care assistant.

1　Is decision-making involved?

2　Is the task carried out frequently?

3　Does the patient require feedback following the task?

4　Is the response to treatment immediate?

5　Are the consequences of error not serious?

Health care professional

Staff nurse

I have to sit down for a good hour to get the care plans sorted, and it is difficult to make sure that everybody has had their care properly. Our care assistants now do so much of the care. We spend time in assessing their apprenticeship units that are about giving care. It is easy to get stuck into management role and actually only do the care plans, the pills, the doctors' rounds and not actually ever wash a patient. Which isn't right, really. Sometimes you don't have a choice and that can be quite upsetting. You know that you just can't be everywhere and you can only do so much, so it's better to support the learning of junior staff.

Interactions between health care professionals, nurses and support staff continue to be affected by the hierarchical structure that operates within clinical settings. Status can be a potential barrier to collegiate decision-making. Whatever the resource problem, it is necessary to remember that 'learning entails giving up old perceptions, comfortable assumptions and states of knowledge or ignorance and draws into question the past approaches, habits and mind-sets of individuals and groups' (Lines and Ricketts, 1994, p.165).

KEY POINTS

● Patient care is considered the priority and this can be viewed as constraining learning through practice.

● Resource issues such as staff shortages can hamper learning

● Circumstances affect learning, because of the opportunities offered (or withheld) by the context.

SPECIALITIES

The different cultures in clinical placements and specialities have been identified by students as having an impact on their learning (Pearcey and Elliott, 2004). Health care students have to learn to adapt to each placement, its characteristics and associated reputations by getting to know staff, and this is helped by having placements of a reasonable length).

Students have been found to go through three phases whilst on placement:

1 adaptation (becoming part of the community)
2 stabilization (increased knowledge and skills)
3 consolidation (requiring reduced supervision) (Crawford and Kiger, 1998).

Reflective activity

What would be the optimum length of placement for a second-year student coming to the area you are presently in? Think about how long (on average) it takes for you to adapt to a new clinical speciality? Have you found any particular area difficult to adapt to, and if so why do you think this was?

Pearcey and Elliott (2004) found some negative attitudes towards longer-stay patients. A fast turnover can limit the amount of time that nurses have to get to know the patients. In Melia's (1987) seminal study, students suggested that 'real nursing' occurred mostly on wards, happened at speed, and involved technical procedures or drug administration. Work described as 'proper nursing' focused on care of younger clients, was done at a fast pace, and feelings of success were measured in cure or discharge (Melia, 1987). It was not just regarded as 'passing the time' as in care of the elderly (Melia, 1987, p. 133). Melia suggests that students took the speciality as a reference point for the value of their own work and their preferences might simply reflect their stage of development as adults and nurses.

A report, by the Commission on Improving Dignity in Care for Older People in 2012 (an Alliance of NHS Confederation, Age UK and Local Government Association), suggests that 'a major cultural shift' is needed in caring for the ageing population and warns that even a few days of poor treatment can have a devastating effect. Older people describe how their skills, self-confidence and ability to look after themselves can deteriorate as a direct result of the way they are treated, such as being spoken to as if they were a child, or having things done to them, rather than with them. Feeding someone just to save time, rather than helping them to eat, can feel humiliating and create dependence, while telling them what to wear or what time to go to bed, robs them of choices and dignity. A deterioration, such as incontinence or immobility, resulting from undignified care can set in extraordinarily quickly. The report calls for a change in NHS hospital services to manage long term conditions with complex co-morbidities rather than diagnosing and treating for single acute illnesses. Older people should be welcomed, valued and have their needs understood and met, for example how they would like to be addressed and staff should challenge discriminatory behaviours, with praise going to those who identify shortcomings. Getting the training right for staff (students and CPD) is important, including dementia care, maintaining dignity and compassion in care, working with patients who have communication deficits. The report says universities and colleges recruiting nursing and medical students should include compassion in their admission criteria, and the ability of new care staff to be respectful should be assessed during a probationary period. Hospital workers should also be given a few minutes at the end of their shift to reflect on how they could do better and relatives who wish to help should not be treated as a nuisance.

Smith's (1992) study also supported the increased prestige attached to technical and mental work. Students were affected by the atmosphere of the clinical area, particularly if nurses were viewed as not making the effort to talk with their patients and build up the nurse–patient relationship (Pearcey and Elliott, 2004). By contrast, when a clinical area had high morale, a positive atmosphere and encouraged staff development, the students were motivated in their continued interest in nursing. The students within Pearcey and Elliott's (2004) study were concerned that so much of their learning through practice came from negative experiences and that, through a need to 'fit in', they too could become socialized into a less caring approach to patients.

EVIDENCE BASE

Read this article: Tucker *et al.* (2006) Physiotherapy students' sources of stress, perceived course difficulty, and paid employment: Comparison between Western Australia and United Kingdom. *Physiotherapy Theory and Practice*, **22**(6): 317–328.
Do you think that learners encounter these challenges in your area?

EMOTIONAL LABOUR

You may, perhaps, take the view that emotions just happen to you and that you are not fully responsible for them; however, they involve a degree of cognition and are also 'socioculturally constituted'. A clinical team's belief systems and values affect the capacity and characteristics of emotional expression. Hochschild (1983), who suggests that 'feeling rules' are socially variable and historically changing, has focused on uncomfortable emotion management within work settings. Staff within clinical settings do find time for 'fun' and humour as this can help them to confront the less enjoyable aspects of practice, develop camaraderie and a sense of community (Castro *et al.*, 1999). Emotional labour required for caring for people in distress is often balanced by emotional release through humour and jokes (Wigens, 2004). Maeve (1998) found that the humorous issues and content of jokes could be considered shocking or inappropriate, if heard by people outside a clinical setting.

Reflective activity

Have you noticed the use of humour within clinical settings to relieve stress? Did this ever concern you, or appear 'inappropriate' when you were on clinical placement or in a new locality?

In the past, nurses were encouraged to appear busy and were advised to maintain a professional barrier to avoid becoming emotionally involved with patients (Menzies, 1960). Concentrating on 'tasks' can detach nurses from feelings and reduce the nurse–patient relationship. Menzies suggested that social structures within nursing, such as the routines of care were a form of defence, to avoid anxiety, guilt, doubts and uncertainty, by denying the significance of the individual. Menzies suggested that it was perhaps the most defensive individuals who stay in nursing and that those unable to cope with the rigidity of the system, the elimination of personal discretion and growth left the profession.

Parsons' (1968) seminal work identified that professional socialization creates affect-neutral practitioners who avoid emotional involvement with clients. James (1992) suggested that in practice individualized care may only amount to finding out enough about patients to know when to interrupt routines to attend to individual requirements. Allen (2000) found that although nurses wanted to involve family and friends in care, implementing this in practice placed additional demands on their limited time. When the management of nursing care results in a requirement to speed-up 'the human assembly line', this makes 'genuine' personal service harder to deliver and it becomes virtually impossible to deliver emotional labour and individualized psychological care (Wigens, 1997).

The claim that there has been movement from the domination of physical care and limited nurse–patient communication to more holistic care is still open to challenge by studies that report similar superficial, task-focused communication (Hewinson, 1999). A number of models (types) of nurse–patient relationships have been identified as below.

Models of practitioner–patient relationships

1 Nurse centred

This emphasized the patient's dependence on the health carer. Care giving was determined by the nurse who was viewed as more 'knowledgeable' than the patient. Care is delivered in the patient's best interest.

2 Technical relationship

Nursing is seen as a clinical science, where skilled technical, objective care is competently delivered without imposing any of the carer's values or wishes. The patient may have the ultimate responsibility for determining needs, but the nurse informs and has current evidence and skills to impart.

3 Patient centred

The nurse works alongside the patient, negotiating the role of the nurse as applicable to the situation and individual patient needs. Within this model, there is the possibility for the nurse and patient to 'know' each other as people.

4 Therapeutic relationship

Therapeutic relationship requires the nurse to respect and have genuine interest in the person, to show emotional warmth, tolerance and non-judgemental acceptance of the patient. It also calls for the practitioner to use 'self' in nursing interactions, whilst maintaining awareness of their limitations and adherence to ethical codes. The patient plays a part in a therapeutic relationship by helping in making decisions about what interventions are right for them and being motivated to understand the treatment/care and their role within this.

Perhaps you identified during the reflective activity that not every patient requires a deep practitioner–patient relationship, but that wherever possible it should be patient centred. Eraut (1994) suggests that there is a close link between client centredness and continuing to develop one's professional knowledge. As nurses and other health care practitioners have started to research and explore the nurse–patient relationship, there has been increasing interest in the concept of emotional labour.

Reflective activity

During your time working in various clinical settings have you seen all of these forms of the nurse–patient relationship? Do you think that patient problems, the length of the patient episode or the age of the patient influenced the nurse–patient relationships observed?

From an emotional labour approach, emotions are brought in line with feeling rules by two means:

- **Surface acting** – in this case, the nurse puts on the expressive visage or body stance of the emotion in the hope of stimulating the authentic feeling, changing feeling from the outside in.

- **Deep acting** – here, more profound strategies, such as imaging and verbal and physical prompting are used, modifying bodily or mental states, changing the feeling from the inside out (Hochschild, 1983). An example of prompts to deep acting might be the way the nurses talk to each other during a handover when they are discussing the care of a dying patient and his or her relatives.

Student nurses have been found to experience anxiety and stress because their emotional labour was largely unrecognized and undervalued, and their workloads meant that there was only time to meet the physical and technical needs of patients (Smith, 1992). The 'little things' of caring were not being recognized or costed in the work environment that emphasized 'getting the work done' and rewarded non-patient-oriented activities (Smith, 1992). The concept of emotional labour helps in understanding how emotions have become a commodity in the work environment, just like technical skills, such as prescribing. Overt examples of lack of caring from senior nursing staff can affect the future working of junior staff, so role models for care giving and emotional labour are important for student nurses.

Reflective activity

With another person, reflect on an incident where you observed an experienced nurse acting as a role model for psychological care giving. What did you particularly notice about their practice?

How did it feel to discuss and share this incident with another person? Reflective learning itself can be seen as a form of emotional labour, as nurses share and work through difficult issues and problems with other nurses.

Nurses working with more insight into the home situation and usual lifestyle of the patient feel that this helps develop patient–nurse relationships. 'Having a picture' of the patient as a person in the world is personal knowledge that affected care delivery (Wigens, 2004). Perhaps this is part of the 'imaging' that Hochschild (1983) suggests is required for 'deep acting'. The length of time and continuity of patient care is seen as a contributory factor in allowing deeper, therapeutic relationships to develop (Wigens, 2004). This has been reinforced within the care of patients with dementia through the use of the 'This is me' tool which provides a 'snapshot' of the person with dementia, giving information about them as an individual, such as needs, preferences, likes, dislikes and interests (Alzheimer's Society, 2012). This enables staff to treat each person as an individual, thereby reducing distress for them and their carers and helping to prevent issues such as malnutrition and dehydration.

Senior nurses within a clinical setting play a crucial role in developing the social construction of emotional work, setting the 'tone' for staff, patients and visitors (Wilson-Barnett *et al.*, 1995). Senior nurses need to be open to new ideas, allow a flexible approach to routines and be supportive to staff so that individualized care can be provided (James, 1992). Lawler (1991) found that 'expert nurses' achieved a fine balance between showing concern and care for the patient whilst also appearing professional. During a working day, various situations require differing degrees of emotional work, and this can range from a minimal level, when giving routine 'basic' care, to a greater level, when caring for a dying patient (Bolton, 2001). Bolton stresses the emotional complexity within nursing work by employing the term 'emotional jugglers' to highlight nurses' capacity to present a variety of faces. Mentors and 'link lecturers' assume a key role for students in learning about emotional work.

When Priest (1999) compared 'expert' and 'novice' understanding of psychological care, she identified that experts considered information giving as a major aspect, whereas novices placed more emphasis upon personal qualities. Experts concentrated on handling emotions and novices focused on facilitating the expression of emotions; Priest (1999) suggested that this is because experts are more mindful that encouraging patients to 'open up' may require time which is unavailable owing to competing demands and priorities. According to Priest (1999), the specific training programmes in psychological care have not been adopted by nurses, as there is some doubt as to whether psychological care can be taught, whether it is solely developed through experience or indeed whether all nurses can develop psychological care-giving abilities. The nurses' own life experiences are seen as integral to their patient care.

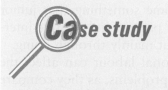

Case study

Emotional labour and patient expectations

A team meeting was being held – led by a senior nurse for the unit – as there had been some complaints regarding the lack of 'caring attitudes' displayed by the nursing staff towards some patients.

The group was split into two smaller discussion groups and the following issues were raised and discussed.

Some nurses said that their critical reflections on practice involved reviewing how much 'feeling' they had integrated into their care giving and that the workload on the ward had reduced the level of this from what they would like to have delivered. Others said that not getting 'too involved' was important and that this formed part of their personal philosophy of care. Both groups agreed that professional working required a balance of personal value judge-ments about how much time to spend with individual patients. One nurse was seen as a role model for caring skills within the ward team, even though she was not one of the most experienced members of staff. She talked about the need to 'give something' of herself as an open and honest 'real person', to build effective patient relationships, but did not feel that this was realistic for all patients within their care.

The ward nurses talked about bringing their per-sonal learning from their home life to their nursing and vice versa. Nurses' personal knowledge from their home life meant that they accepted that they 'made contact' with certain patients only, and with others they were only likely to develop superficial relationships. There was a process of selecting the depth of involvement with individual patients, which related to the priorities within the clinical area at the time. There was consensus that emotional involve-ment with a patient and relatives was demanding but can also make a role feel more worthwhile. The staff had been very upset about the complaints about their caring communications.

What suggestions do you think could help these ward staff work on this aspect of their practice? How might they manage their caring and emotional labour to meet their patients' expectations?

Students learn to 'tune into' the emerging priorities within a placement and to calls for situated understanding of the emotional labour requirements. Student nurses accumulated knowledge of emotional labour through experi-ence and were able to talk reflectively about nursing experience with staff and colleagues. Most nurses expect their psychological care and empathy to develop through trial-and-error learning, the passage and exposure of prac-tice, observation of role models and feedback from patients, with reflective diaries or portfolios assisting this process (Priest, 1999).

Increasing nursing experience does not necessarily equate with improved communication and psychological caring (Wigens, 2004). The circumstances when nurses are more likely to become 'personally close' with patients include when patients are critically or acutely ill, suffering psychological distress, dying, angry and aggressive, or when the patient or situation closely mirrors people or situations from the nurses' personal lives (Wigens, 2004). It can prove difficult for students to observe 'emotionally challenging situations' as an observational role may affect the dynamics of a difficult clinical situa-tion. This aspect of practice, therefore, has become something that junior nurses learn through observation of fragments of patient and relative inter-actions, and discussions with experienced staff, but mainly through doing.

The constant requirement to undertake emotional labour can affect the meaning that nurses attach to their own personal problems, as they compare their own issues to those of patients within their care, and this meant that they viewed them from a different perspective (Wigens, 2004). Interactions (formal and informal, social and professional contact during work hours) between nurses and colleagues are viewed as important to supporting caring, and nurses generally indicate a high level of satisfaction with these. Informal support networks often comprise other nurses who play a crucial role in maintaining stability by making themselves available to discuss a distressing clinical situation (Wigens, 2004). In order to make professional judgements in an emotionally charged situation, nurses learn to vent their personal feelings later, after the event (Wigens, 2004). A sign of nursing maturity was that, even though 'some part of a difficult incident' remains with the nurse, they avoid bringing this home (Wigens, 2004). Nurses use their emotions on a daily basis in their practice, selecting the depth and level of their emotional work.

SERVICE IMPROVEMENT

A fundamental change in thinking, practice and delivery of health care has been called for to build a health service around the needs of the patient alongside ambitious plans to make the health service a better place to work. The continuous drive to improve the quality of care that is delivered seems a logical aim for any registered health care practitioner, this culture influences the learning environment. Moving to patient led rather than 'doing to and for', working with patients. Modernization and transformation of care pathways have become a key driver, workforce issues focus on a steady improvement in productivity and quality, and good systematic management and organizational development.

The NHS Institute of Innovation and Improvement was formed to support the NHS with high impact solutions to some of the biggest challenges, its mission including accelerating the uptake of proven innovation. In 2010 the 'Equity and Excellence – Liberating the NHS' white paper (Department of Health 2010c) was released as the British government felt that although the NHS was a great institution founded on important principles it could be better for patients and staff. This set the vision for the future of the NHS. The NHS Institute for Innovation and Improvement (2009) has identified five frames with which to inspire change: they are:

- Performance and Health
- The Discovery process
- The Influence model
- Change Architecture
- The benefits hierarchy

They discuss the need for creating 'healthy' organizations and systems which will deliver performance tomorrow and the day after, changing mindsets, wider ranging, well sequenced initiatives covering broad perspectives of change which have robust performance measurement strategies. With factors such as an ageing population putting the NHS under increasing pressure, and the global economic pressures being faced, it is not possible to go on as before. The NHS has to achieve value for money and the best possible quality so that patients get the greatest benefit (DoH, 2010d). The Quality, Innovation, Productivity and Prevention (QIPP) programme is all about ensuring that each pound spent is used to bring maximum benefit and quality of care to patients: DoH has set up twelve workstreams to help manage the delivery of QIPP in the NHS (DoH, 2010d). The national workstreams fit into three key areas; commissioning and pathways, provider efficiency and system enablers.

Transformation of health services requires a breaking down of traditional barriers to find new and flexible ways of thinking and doing, calling for creative responses. Implicit within service improvement is the ability to change, develop new roles, interprofessional working, lifelong learning and collegiate working (Gough, 2001). Service improvement can place additional demands on nurses, requiring them to implement change whilst still having to complete the ongoing clinical care. Many health carers are sceptical about the finance available for properly supporting modernization and there is a perception that managers are more concerned with finance than they are with patient care (Callaghan, 2003; Wigens, 2004). The relentless pursuit of quality is combined with the need to meet financial challenges as never before. For example, the NHS in order to meet significant additional demand will need to fund new technologies and drugs, this involves making efficiency savings of up to £20 billion (DoH, 2011), at the same time as driving up quality.

The changes required to implement evidence-based practice can sometimes tip the fine balance of everyday coping, where much of this practice is based on tacit knowledge, sometimes made explicit through reflection. Change, even when acknowledged as improving patient care, can overload and stretch clinical staff who have 'learnt to manage'. Modernization within nursing has lead to the ownership and co-ordination of patient flow, and patient flow can become the management of people into bed spaces rather than seeing patients as individuals. Nursing teams adapt their working to help 'meet a target', implement evidence-based change (Heitlinger, 1999) and empower patients, in such a way that change is minimized (Wigens, 2004).

Clinical teams who feel a sense of 'change overload' more easily accept change if patient care is improved as an outcome. The overall success of a change can also be dependent on whether nurses feel that the nursing team has ownership of the change. Colleagues are easily accessible and able to adapt messages to counter individual, organizational and environmental barriers and are able to harness multiple approaches to changing practice, including one-to-one educational approaches, influencing clinical audit agendas, clinical teaching, mentorship and role modelling.

Over to you

Find out about the service improvement structure within your organization. Have you been involved in any initiatives such as the productive ward series?

Look at **www.institute.nhs.uk** there are many different opportunities available.

Modernization has led to the development of expanded roles and the re-engineering of nursing roles (Tye and Ross, 2000). Service improvements can be a route for career diversity for nurses and other health care professions, such as specialist, advanced practitioner and consultant roles that add to the highly differentiated careers. New roles increase opportunities for retaining and developing senior nurses, raising the profile of the profession, without the overall caring motivations being lost (Callaghan, 2003). Opposition to the medicalization of nurses' role and identity and to potential de-skilling competes alongside the increased professional and career opportunities (Tye and Ross, 2000). Perceived inequities in workload between general and specialist staff can occur along with a blurring of the distinct or unique differences between nursing and medicine. New roles within nursing inevitably create uncertainty owing to the reconstructing of professional identity (Williams and Sibbald, 1999). Nurse practitioners and specialist nurses can feel a sense of isolation from the rest of the nursing staff, made tangible through different uniforms and different geographical locations (Tye and Ross, 2000). Foucault (1972) believed that it is through discourse that the social production of meaning occurs and that power and knowledge are inextricably linked. Specialization has probably gained power and legitimacy from its knowledge base; however, by the very process of differentiation and the establishment and maintenance of distinct identities, it can lead to reduced collaboration and to tribalism.

Over to you

Find out about the specialist practitioner roles that visit or link with your current clinical area. Take opportunities to learn through practice by shadowing one of these staff for a shift or during a patient interaction. Discuss their role and what knowledge underpins their practice.

Armstrong and Armstrong (1996) argue that there is a growing fragmentation of nursing work due to the hegemony of the medical model, with tasks being reassigned to different categories of nurses.

Increased standardization and the use of information technology means that some nurses perceive that the requirement for professional judgement and autonomy has been reduced, and inflexible barriers are being created (Wigens, 2004). However, the introduction of new technology can also create an opportunity for learning. New technologies are more accepted if they have a direct impact on workload, but the initial time taken to learn about new equipment must 'pay back' quickly through improved patient care in order for a clinical team to continue investing time in training (Wigens, 2004).

Hegemony
An organizing principle or common-sense ideology that permeates throughout society and is socialized into everyday life and accepted by the majority

EVIDENCE BASE

Have a look at some of the information on these websites:

● www.nhsdirect.nhs.uk

● www.connectingforhealth.nhs.uk

● www.institute.nhs.uk

How have technology and the increased access to information influenced learning through practice?

Student nurses have been found to have a deficit in their knowledge of how to effectively improve clinical practice, involving the management of change, even though this should be embedded in all health care professional training. Reflection mainly takes a written form submitted to a lecturer, and students want to be given feedback on their reflection whilst in the clinical setting (Kyrkjebø and Hage, 2005). There is a mismatch between what students learn about quality patient care and what they actually observe in practice. Kyrkjebø and Hage, who used a focus group methodology with a sample of 27 Norwegian student nurses, suggest that there is a need to encourage reflection and openness to allow students to scrutinize why errors and omissions in care occur.

Improvement of knowledge and processes can be separated into four elements:

● knowledge of the organizational system in which health care is delivered and of how involved patients are in making decisions about care

● knowledge of the variation in processes, products and people and how to measure this

● knowledge of accountability, psychology and social working and the approach to change

● knowledge of how to link theory to action so that the knowledge becomes locally useful (Batalden and Stoltz, 1993).

The development of improvement knowledge can be helped by learning the 'plan–do–study–act' (PDSA) cycle (Batalden and Stoltz, 1993) (see Figure 9.2).

The PDSA cycle gives a systematic way of developing new knowledge through learning by experience. However, some health professionals seem to lack the ability to see health care delivery as a process which can be identified, mapped, measured and studied for variation (Mohammed, 2004). An environment that harnesses the PDSA cycle and encourages thinking about 'working smarter' needs to be supported. Nursing can be viewed as 'doing', rather than also about talking and discussing. Time to discuss and plan service

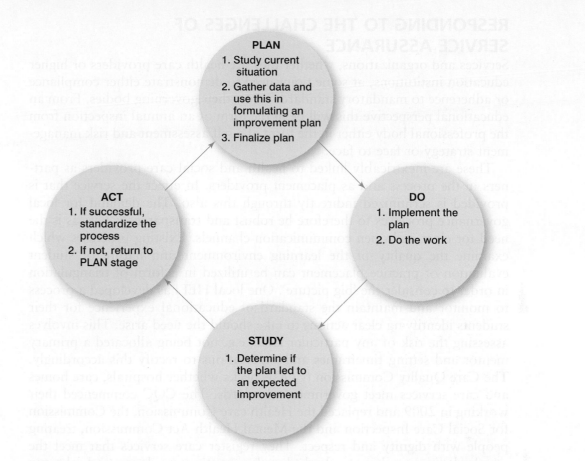

Figure 9.2   PDSA cycle, (adapted from Batalden and Stoltz, 1993)

improvement changes should be balanced alongside 'doing' within clinical environments and is a crucial facet in learning through practice.

Pre-registration learners will encounter the model for service improvement at some point during their programmes so will seek the support of their mentors in identifying examples from practice, look to practitioners as role models for their creative ideas and the implementation of evidence-based practice.

Reflective activity

Think about your area of practice. Is there something that to you seems very simple or obvious that would have an impact on your service users outcome. Add value to their experience but also ensure that resources are more appropriately used? It may be something that you do every day that you could improve but don't know where to start. Small ideas can make a big difference!

RESPONDING TO THE CHALLENGES OF SERVICE ASSURANCE

Services and organizations, whether they are health care providers or higher education institutions, at some point need to demonstrate either compliance or adherence to mandatory standards set by their governing bodies. From an educational perspective this will be in the form of an annual inspection from the professional body either in the form of a self assessment and risk management strategy or face to face.

These are inextricably linked to health and social care providers as partners in the process and as placement providers. In effect the service that is provided is scrutinized indirectly through this also. The demand for local governance processes to therefore be robust and transparent is key, as is the need for clear and open communication channels. Existing processes which examine the quality of the learning environment and nature of student evaluation of practice placement can be utilized in a form of triangulation in order to consider the 'big picture'. One local HEI has developed a process to monitor and maintain the standard of educational experience for their students identifying clear actions to take should the need arise. This involves assessing the risk of any particular issue, e.g. not being allocated a primary mentor and setting timeframes and expectations to rectify this accordingly. The Care Quality Commission (CQC) checks whether hospitals, care homes and care services meet government standards. The CQC commenced their working in 2009 and replaced the Health care Commission, the Commission for Social Care Inspection and the Mental Health Act Commission, treating people with dignity and respect. They register care services that meet the standards, inspect them to check that they continue to do so, and take any remedial action when standards are not met. These standards include making sure food and drink meets people's needs; making sure that the environment is clean and safe; managing and staffing services. Inspectors visit organizations to check they are meeting the standards and carry out unannounced inspections of services on a regular basis and in response to concerns raised (CQC, 2012).

Nurses are in an important position to lead and motivate their teams to improve care and identify and address any shortfalls (Young, 2009). Practitioners play a major role in all aspects of quality patient care management, however the frequency with which new policies and directives are being published can be overwhelming (Glasper, 2010a). Having said this, ensuring that standards are met through regular monitoring is now a part of everyday practice and evident in governance processes.

THE LEARNING ORGANIZATION

The Audit Commission (2001) suggests that it is necessary to engender a culture that values and expects training, learning and development. Billions of pounds are spent yearly on learning and professional development of health care staff in the NHS so there needs to be sound justification for investing in continuing professional development (CPD). The quality of education is now being judged on its impact on practitioners' ability to deliver health services as part of a flexible competent workforce. The importance of getting health professional education 'right' is an area of continuing debate. Levett-Jones (2005) suggests that CPD not only enhances knowledge and skills but there is also a positive correlation between professional development and staff satisfaction, staff retention and quality patient care. Nurses' ability to gain access to lifelong learning activities is aligned to retention in the clinical setting and, therefore, improved staffing levels. Mackereth (1989) found that staff felt valued if they had access to CPD and that this affected their morale, motivation and wish to stay within practice.

Over to you

Locate and read a study-leave policy.

Speak to three qualified staff health professional staff and ask them what training, education and continuous professional activities they have been involved with during the last year. Were there any differences in their ability to access CPD activities? If so, what were the reasons and how do you think this situation could be improved?

Study-leave policies need to be developed in consultation with staff, managers and professional bodies, and it is necessary to meet legal and statutory requirements. Managers should be made aware of the cost and significance of mistakes, in terms of education, training and development decisions, and how these mistakes can affect long- and short-term organizational priorities. An organization's policy should aim to gain maximum benefit from education, and the policy should, therefore, identify priorities, encourage equity of training opportunities and give guidance to managers who are agreeing personal development plans. This can mean, however, that staff only have access to education that is regarded as organizationally high-priority; so one method used by some organizations for linking personal and organizational educational planning has been to offer annual credits for funding flexibility.

Increasing access to education and development is important, and guidelines for determining individual, directorate and Trust access to study leave should be transparent. Opportunities for education and training vary among different NHS Trusts (Audit Commission, 2001). Finding the time to undertake CPD activities can often be the biggest issue affecting access by health care professionals (Simons and Parry-Crooke, 2001). In one case site, there was variability in access to CPD activities between differing specialities within the same organization (Wigens, 2004); this appeared to be linked to staffing levels and to the value placed on CPD by nurse leaders.

Training involves the systematic development of the knowledge, skills and attitudes required by an individual to perform a task or job adequately. An education strategy includes the processes for education and training within the workplace, which are regularly undertaken by an employing organization, and should identify the way that education and training will be implemented, evaluated and audited over time. The strategy should link education and training activities to the priorities identified through business planning within the organization (see Figure 9.3).

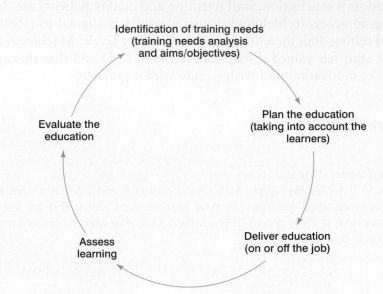

Figure 9.3   Education cycle

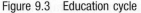

Range of factors driving an education strategy

The identification and analysis of training needs:

- Finance availability (scarce resources can be targeted, e.g. replacement finance for staff)
- New developments in the service
- The costs of study programmes (travel)
- Identification of available education (off the job) or the need for the creation of new education programmes based on learning objectives
- Format for the education, e.g. on the job – demonstration, coaching, rotation (planned experience), assignments or projects
- Improvements in staff knowledge and skills that are required
- The identification of key people who will be able to attend (can the education be interprofessional?)
- What benefits will be gained from the experience/education?
- How will staff pass on their knowledge and skills?
- Realistic timescales for completion

In transforming services there will also be a need to modernize health care roles. This requires an organization to have a broad span of activities in place to aid recruitment and retention, including mentorship, preceptorship and clinical supervision training, return to practice, apprenticeship training, flexible retirement, incentives and improved work practices. Healthy working conditions and an organizational culture where employees feel valued and have a common sense of loyalty, can enhance retention of staff. By supporting a range of lifelong learning, an organization can signal the value attached to learning.

A Training Needs Analysis (TNA) informs decision-making and is part of an education strategy. A TNA gives a baseline set of data to identify priorities and provides feedback on the effectiveness of previous decisions. Through the TNA:

- Learning objectives are established.
- Knowledge is mapped.
- Gaps are identified.
- Appropriate action is taken.
- Organizational issues are considered e.g. clinical developments.
- Data may be collected through questionnaires, observation, interviews and staff records.

Training needs analysis can be undertaken for an organization as a whole, for departments or teams, or for individuals (sometimes the latter is called learning needs assessment [LNA]). Learning needs assessment is a part of TNA that assesses and understands an individual's needs through personal development planning (discussed within Chapter 5). Skilled contracting practices by Trusts, using best available data, assist organizations and their local education providers in ensuring that appropriate spending on education is targeted towards local priorities and staff needs.

The three basic methods for analyzing education needs are:

- surveys and questionnaires to staff
- job analysis linked to the requirements for the job (e.g. KSF profile)
- personal development plan reviews.

The processes of TNA and LNA can be time consuming, and it can prove difficult to target specific areas, so the responsibility for delivering the education strategy is not just the employer's, but also the individual employee's. It is important that education is evaluated not only by seeing whether the objectives for the individual and the service area have been met but also whether the overall purpose has been achieved.

Kirkpatrick (1975) suggests that there are four levels of evaluation that can be undertaken with regard to education:

1 **reaction** – how the participants felt about the education; can be obtained through discussion, an evaluation sheet or questionnaire

2 **learning** – determining what skills and knowledge have been learnt through assessment

3 **behaviour** – observing the application of learning within the workplace

4 **results** – determining the effect on the organization or the department of the education.

Reflective activity

Consider some education that you have received; this can be on or off the job. What was your immediate reaction to the education? What skills or knowledge did you gain as a result of this education that could be used in your practice? What level of evaluation was undertaken with regard to this education?

Health care provider organizations should be lifelong learning organizations, making use of every opportunity to develop their staff, strengthening the image of the organization as a 'good' employer. For example, there could be a structured plan for developing leadership skills throughout the organization. The overall education, training and development strategy should reflect changes in work practices, team and individual needs, and local as well as national issues.

An organization's culture refers to it's learned beliefs, values, norms, symbols and traditions that are common to them. These shared qualities make it unique (Handy, 1999). The culture is about the ways of working and behaving, each organization is different. However Handy (1999) suggests that a culture cannot be precisely defined it is something that is perceived, this infers a subjective element. There may be different cultures within an organization. Senge (2006) identifies five basic steps toward becoming a learning organization:

1 Systems thinking

2 Team building

3 Personal mastery

4 Mental models

5 Building a shared vision

Application of these principles and learning skills allows for the creation of teamwork within the organization, they create a motivating environment for team learning, individual growth as well as business growth. Whilst students are supernumerary they nevertheless do contribute to the care delivered by engaging in service user activities, and as such affect and are affected by the organizational and unit culture (Levett-Jones and Lathlean, 2009). Having agreed organization-wide values this can be the basis for cultural change, with staff recruitment, promotion and appraisal being based on these values. We will explore how strategies to lead learning can be developed in the online bonus feature to accompany this chapter.

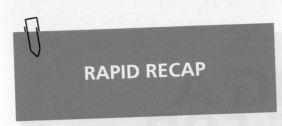

RAPID RECAP

Check your progress so far by working through each of the following questions.

1 What strategies may nurses use to cope with high workloads, time pressures and information overload?

2 What three phases do Crawford and Kiger (1998) suggest students progress through whilst on clinical placement?

3 Outline the main aspects of the four models of practitioner–patient relationship.

4 What is meant by the term 'emotional labour'?

5 What do the letters PDSA stand for in the service improvement cycle?

6 How might a multidisciplinary team that could be described as 'committed' (Bruce, 1980) show that they are working interprofessionally?

If you have difficulty with any of these questions, read through the section again to refresh your understanding before moving on.

FURTHER READING

Theodosisus, C. (2008) *Emotional Labour in Health care: The unmanaged heart of nursing.* Routledge. London.

CHAPTER 10

CREATING A CLIMATE FOR LEARNING

LEARNING OBJECTIVES

By the end of this chapter you should be able to:

- explain your professional code/guidelines for practice placements

- critically assess and evaluate a clinical area as a learning environment

- appreciate ways of getting the most from clinical environments, e.g. hub and spoke, teaching and learning programmes

- explain the main curricula changes that have occurred within health professional education

- value the range of educational roles that support learning through practice

- recognize how higher education institutes and service providers need to work together to optimize learning through practice.

Bonus features for this chapter available on the book's website

INTRODUCTION

In this, the final chapter, we look at clinical placements, and clinical settings in general, to work out what issues impact on learning through practice. Health care professional students work in a variety of clinical settings, and individual experiences can affect perceptions of different specialities and different professions. The aim is for you to appreciate the importance of formal and informal learning within clinical settings.

You will gain an awareness of how the learning climate within a clinical setting is affected by changing curricula and policy implementation. Although much of the discussion looks at nursing, professional education within nursing mirrors that of many health care professions, for example physiotherapy, dietetics. The chapter explores key educational roles not based solely within clinical settings, including practice educators, link lecturers and professional and practice development roles, and stresses the importance of academic and service partnership working. This chapter brings together many of the themes that you encountered within previous chapters and that contribute to developing effective communities of practice within clinical placements.

THE CLINICAL LEARNING ENVIRONMENT

All learners and staff within clinical areas are adults. Having a concept of the adult learner (defined as andragogy and discussed in Chapter 2) may help in thinking about a particular clinical learning environment. Students' level of satisfaction is raised when they are treated with respect and as individuals (Randle, 2003). Students' needs should be considered within a well-managed and motivated clinical learning situation.

CLINICAL CASE LOAD

Answer the following questions about your current clinical area to determine the clinical teaching caseload and to assess the area as a clinical learning environment; where appropriate, identify action points.

1 Give a brief description of the practical experience offered in this area.

2 Is practice supported by high standards of documentation regarding client/patient care/treatment?

3 Are clinical governance arrangements in place to support evidence-based practice?

4 Is the environment physically, socially and psychologically safe for staff and clients/patients?

5 Are all mentors/supervisors familiar with the assessment strategy of students' courses?

6 Do mentors/supervisors get the opportunity to meet and work regularly with their students?

7 Are there sufficient mentors/supervisors to ensure appropriate levels of supervision? (Has the maximum number of students the area can supervise been identified, and the number of staff who are fully prepared for a supervision role?)

8 Are there effective communication channels between staff and clients?

9 Are local policies/guidelines/protocols accessible and up to date?

10 Do students receive a 'welcome pack'/orientation on arrival in the area?

11 Do you receive formal and informal evaluations of the learning environment from students?

12 Does the practice experience enable students to gain experience of the role of qualified staff in a range of contexts?

13 Do students gain experience of working interprofessionally?

14 Is the clinical team spirit motivated towards developing students' learning?

15 What learning/facilitation roles are available for students, e.g. mentor/preceptor/clinical supervisor; practice educator; teacher/lecturer/tutor; others?

Question 14 asked you to assess the clinical team spirit. Team spirit does impact on the overall learning environment (Wigens, 2004). However, it is important to remember that a popular placement is not necessarily synonymous with an effective learning environment, although there are obvious advantages.

Health care professional

Registered practitioner

Being a placement area for senior third year students helps recruitment, both in a sense of bringing would-be employees into close contact with the team and so encouraging them to apply for vacancies. It also provides a hands-on opportunity for us to experience the work of the would-be applicants.

Having started to identify the strengths and weaknesses in the clinical area in which you are presently working, it is perhaps useful to see what researchers have found out about the vital elements for good placement learning experiences. Papp *et al.* (2003) and Koh (2002), researching in Finland and England respectively, found that there needed to be high levels of co-operation between staff members, enhanced care standards, and a good atmosphere where students are regarded as colleagues. Students wanted to feel appreciated for their contribution to clinical practice and to feel part of the team, and their supervisor/mentor is vital in assisting with this. The clinical setting is often changing and sometimes unpredictable, which can make it hard to plan an optimal clinical learning environment for students. Even so, from your previous review of the learning environment, you can probably identify some areas for improvement.

Over to you

Improvement action plan:

● Having thought about your current workplace/placement as a learning environment, what would be the first thing you would do to bring about improvements?

● Draw up a list of achievable steps aimed at prioritizing and implementing your improvements.

It is essential that arrangements are made to ensure that issues of diversity are taken into account, for instance ethnicity, disability and gender are thought about during the placement, so that there is evidence that the requirements of equal opportunities/equalities policies are met on an ongoing basis.

Health care professionals can bemoan the lack of time for teaching in clinical settings, and, when evaluating a clinical placement, students sometimes say that they have learnt little because there were no formal teaching sessions. These perceptions of learning fail to acknowledge that a stimulating clinical environment allows a great deal of informal learning to take place. Even so, effective learning in clinical practice does require the structured management of the following:

1 identifying learning needs
2 specifying learning objectives
3 determining available learning resources, experiences and strategies
4 agreeing evidence of accomplishment of learning objectives
5 specifying how the evidence will be validated
6 reviewing and assessing learning
7 evaluating the learning environment.

STRUCTURING CLINICAL LEARNING

The first clinical placement has a powerful influence on confirming the health care career choice made by a student. Recognizing the importance of a structured approach to practice learning can, therefore, be influential in retaining students.

EVIDENCE BASE

Read: Chesser-Smyth, P. (2005) The lived experiences of general student nurses on their first clinical placement: A phenomenological study. *Nurse Education in Practice*, 5, 320–7.

Through in-depth interviews with nursing students in Ireland, Chesser-Smyth found that:

Although the initial observation stage (on a first placement) appears to last approximately two weeks, it was only when students became actively involved in the workload together with the acquisition of new knowledge that confidence levels increased and anxiety reduced.

Chesser-Smyth, 2005, p. 326

Many students may experience **reality shock** (Kramer, 1974) when they move out of the skills laboratories into clinical areas, and students may feel that they need to relearn skills. The stages of reality shock have been defined by Kramer in the following way:

1 Honeymoon – the student is fascinated with the new work.
2 Shock/Rejection – the student rejects the new environment, or the old environment, or self and may become socially isolated.

Reality shock

The conflict caused by the movement from the familiar higher education environment to the unfamiliar work setting, caused by a gap between what has been learnt and on-the-job experiences

3 Recovery – the student is able to see the funny side of this, and is becoming competent.

4 Resolution – the student is able to display culturally appropriate reactions.

Added to this, students often compare their own practice with that of more experienced nurses, and this reinforces a lack of confidence in their own abilities.

Professional confidence

Clinical educators identify role-modelling, discussion, commitment and mutual respect as key ways of promoting confidence, whereas students suggest that encouragement, goodwill, acting as a resource/role model and promoting patient care are important (Flagler *et al.*, 1988). Professional confidence is thought to underpin clinical competency (Bell *et al.*, 1998) and a positive change in the confidence of nursing students has a significant impact on their performance within practice (Farrand *et al.*, 2006). Crooks *et al.* (2005) noted that students developed their professional confidence through becoming informed, finding a voice of their own to discuss their clinical practice, becoming self-directed in their learning and by comparing their care delivery with that of other colleagues at work. Confident mentors/supervisors who are comfortable with supporting, challenging and extending students' learning, and are available to supervise regularly, are the basis of good-quality practice teaching. The work area needs to appreciate the practice teaching component within a practitioner's workload and the time that undertaking this role requires.

Learning needs are identified by the gap between where the learner is presently and where they want to be. This may involve analyzing the skills and knowledge required in performing a particular task or job and identifying where the person stands at the moment in relation to the level of knowledge and skills. Resources required to carry this out should be identified, and steps on the way to achieving the learning outcomes can be agreed. In some clinical settings, this takes the form of a learning contract. A learning contract is an individualized learning plan that should be negotiated between the mentor/supervisor and the learner. It specifies what the student will learn, the time span, how learning will be achieved, and the criteria for measuring success. Using a learning contract hands over the control of learning to the student and modifies the power relations between the assessor and the student. It is important that the learner and mentor/supervisor identify what the learner should be able to demonstrate to show achievement of the learning outcomes. What this evidence looks like then becomes the specific focus of the placement/clinical learning.

Opportunities need to be provided for students to observe safely, rehearse and demonstrate these skills. A variety of methods, including experiential and practice-based learning are employed by the mentor/supervisor to guide the student towards competence. Experiences in practice settings require effective facilitation to meet the desired learning outcomes. To try to help with the structuring of the learning opportunity during a clinical placement, it can be useful to think about the five main approaches to this:

- clinical work with a mentor/supervisor/other
- observing the practice of experienced practitioners
- researching an evidence base for practice in the placement
- a learning pack related to the clinical setting
- thinking of the placement area as a 'hub' and arranging 'spoke' experiences, e.g. visits to other departments, spending time with specialist clinicians (Channell, 2002).

Health care professions are practice-based disciplines and so learning occurs primarily in clinical settings with qualified practitioners acting as role models. Skills and values are projected and learnt, largely subconsciously, during practitioners' everyday work. Clinical teaching is, therefore, an integral part of the qualified professionals' role. Fundamental and specific skills to be developed to improve clinical teaching include the following:

Fundamental clinical teaching skills

- Relationship building
- Negotiating learning contracts
- Questioning
- Active listening
- Challenging
- Reflection skills
- Preparation for learning
- Support skills
- Catalytic skills
- Giving information and advice
- Giving feedback

Look back to Chapter 7 where there is further discussion regarding these skills.

Health care professionals are often inherently good teachers and communicators. They spend a great deal of time teaching patients, family, support staff and other health care professionals. Teaching students in the clinical situation is an aspect of professional development; it requires refining of those teaching skills to cover a variety of scenarios. A short description of a clinical learning situation is included here for you to reflect on the 'key learning issues'. There are no 'correct' answers, but this activity should help you to examine your opinions and values regarding teaching and learning in the clinical environment.

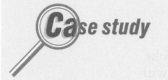

Case study

Welcoming and orientating a student to a new clinical area

The student arrives on the first day of the placement. She has not visited the area beforehand and only has the name of the mentor, whom she approaches. The mentor, standing with arms folded, says that she was not expecting any new student today, but that's not untypical for the way the higher education institute arranges allocations. The mentor suggests that the student settles in by watching how things are done as it is very busy today.

1   How would you have felt if you were this student?

2   Whose responsibility is it in your clinical area to plan a student's orientation?

3   What could the mentor have done to get the placement off to a better start? Identify the negative non-verbal behaviours.

4   In what ways do non-verbal behaviours from a mentor or clinical supervisor affect a student's behaviours and thinking processes?

Having thought about the initial welcome that a student receives from a mentor or supervisor on their first day in a new practice setting, you may have formed a concept of the key facets of a structured and competent orientation meeting. Orientation days, if designed well can reduce student anxiety associated with concerns about lack of skills and knowledge, helps focus on learning outcomes and contribute to fitting in (Worral, 2007). According to Ali and Panther (2008) a good learning environment is one in which students are treated with respect as adult learners, recognizing experience and fostering responsibility for learning. Anecdotal evidence suggests that this reception has a significant impact on the learner's motivation.

Competence includes a broad range of knowledge, attitudes and observable patterns of behaviour which together form the ability to deliver a specified professional service. Many ways have been tried to undertake assessment of clinical skills including:

- simulation
- video testing
- objective structured clinical examination (OSCE)
- observation during 'real practice'.

Obviously, within the placement environment the key feature is the ability to observe and deliver 'real' practice. Students learn in the 'real situation', where the theory they have learnt becomes 'meaningful'. Indeed, when considering learning skills for practice, some theorists suggest that 'skills can only be learnt as an integrated whole in the clinical environment' (Eraut, 1994). This is one example of why the learning that takes place in practice is so important. Clinical areas are busy and, although mentors and supervisors work with students, there are occasions when students may work with unqualified staff or on their own because clinical areas are often short staffed. A supernumerary learner can find it challenging to feel that they are perceived as such when appearing to be part of the team. It is important to recognize and offer assurances to them. This makes learning clinical skills difficult at times.

One conceptual model suggested for promoting learning in clinical contexts is the 'Partner, Learn, Progress' model (Henderson et al., 2006). Within this model, the terms indicate the following:

- Partner – the positive, trusting relationship developed between an experienced practitioner and the learner. Although this is at an interpersonal level, this will be affected by the broader social context, such as the clinical team.

- Learn – the experienced practitioner helps the learner to make sense of all the forms of knowledge that inform practice decisions and delivery: knowledge that may have seemed to the learner to be distant from practice. This mutual collaboration assists the learner in practising safely within the context, making connections between meanings, experiences, feelings and attitudes.

- Progress – the previous two components of the model allow the learner (and the experienced practitioner) to develop their knowledge further.

All students are allocated a named mentor/supervisor who should have appropriate experience of their working environments and meet the necessary requirements as set out by the appropriate professional governing bodies. Mentors/supervisors should guide students for a length of time that is sufficient to enable them to make an informed judgement about students' performance and achievement.

Whenever a mentor/supervisor meets a learner it is useful to structure the meeting appropriately. An example of a possible framework is given below.

TOP TIPS

Framework for meeting with a learner:

1 Think about the introduction and purpose of the meeting

2 Take time to put the learner at ease

3 Explain how the meeting will be recorded

4 Ask generally about how it is going

5 Ask about their practice learning, work/study patterns and if they have any problems

6 Review their assessment work so far

7 Deal with any specific issues the learner wants to raise

8 Discuss the arrangements for follow-up/further meetings

Normally the student and mentor/supervisor should have at least three formal meetings during a clinical placement; guidance for the content of these is given below.

Content of formal meetings

Initial meeting

- To identify the student's learning needs.
- To discuss the learning opportunities available to the student.
- To identify the knowledge and skills available for practice development and assessment.

The student and mentor/supervisor should leave the meeting with enough information to develop their plans, which will be reviewed at the interim/midpoint meeting.

Midpoint meeting

- To review the student's progress in relation to the learning outcomes/plan.
- To identify areas where the student is progressing well and is expected to achieve.
- To identify areas where the student is not progressing as expected and to develop a further action plan to support the student's additional learning needs.

The mentor/supervisor should determine whether additional support should be sought, e.g. clinical placement facilitator, link lecturer.

Final assessment meeting

- To assess the student's overall performance, in relation to the learning outcomes and grading criteria.
- To evaluate the clinical placement learning.

The meeting should be handled in such a way that there is closure. Even though this may not be done on the final placement attendance this should be planned for the final week.

A 'critical mass' of placements and assessors appears to be an important factor in sustaining health care programmes over time. Those employers who are able to offer large numbers of placements on a regular basis often have large numbers of assessors and experienced staff. If a placement has few assessors, the student may be assessed using a 'long-arm' approach where an off-site assessor oversees the assessment by working with the staff who supervise directly, on site.

Health care professional

Link lecturer

We work on the principle that those who can practise can also clinically teach. Associate mentors/supervisors help with student support, assisting the qualified mentors/supervisors so there is almost a team approach to student support. These associate mentors offer support ranging from individual supervision, through joint assessment of the student, to 'arm's length' support as a member of the team. This model allows us to offer 'apprenticeships' to inexperienced assessors who want to develop their skills, as well as allowing other members of the multidisciplinary team to have involvement in the supervision of students from other health care professions. In this way we successfully create a large pool of mentors/assessors.

Lecturers may visit the clinical placement areas, although this varies depending on the health care programme. When a visit does occur, the purpose is mainly to establish that the students feel comfortable in the work setting and have access to the appropriate clinical experiences, and this should be established in a private conversation with the students. The visit also gives the opportunity for the placement staff to let the lecturer know whether they are happy with the placement arrangements, to discuss student performance and to identify any difficulties or issues that have arisen.

TOP TIPS

Top tips for mentors/supervisors:

- Assess your feelings about working with students
- Find out about the students with whom you are working
- Learn to combine giving care and teaching students at the same time
- When it is quiet, offer alternative learning experiences
- Communicate effectively and involve other colleagues, lecturers and practice educators
- Share the important characteristics of your practice, and how you make your clinical decisions with students

LEARNER RESPONSIBILITIES ON PLACEMENT

Overall, learning environments are viewed positively if students are encouraged to take responsibility for their own learning outcomes and are given protected learning time to achieve these. A student has responsibility to be proactive about their learning. Clinical staff can assist by answering questions but they will find it difficult and unrewarding to continue to give information if the student shows little interest. Mentors can assist students to prepare themselves by identifying appropriate texts for pre-placement reading about the clinical speciality and thinking about their needs in relation to the placement and to their stage of training. This will help them to reflect on the experience at a later date. Staff in clinical areas deal with many students and cannot be expected to remember all of an individual student's needs at a particular point in the student's training, especially in areas where there is a very fast throughput of patients. So students need to remind staff if they require a particular experience to achieve their learning outcomes.

An action plan is simply a list of things to be achieved, identifying how this will be done. Although it is common for supervisors to set objectives for learners, learners can also set objectives for themselves. It can help when writing these to begin by stating, 'After this experience/placement I will be able to ...' and then specify what will have been learnt. A set of objectives can also provide a valuable aid to reflection and self-assessment after the placement.

In addition, students need to perceive that their learning experiences are equitable in comparison with those of other students, and that they have received the appropriate mix of support and supervision from experienced and knowledgeable members of the multidisciplinary team.

Student

The supervisor on my last placement was really helpful in making sure that I had the experiences I needed as a student, asking me specifically if there was something I wanted to do that I hadn't done yet. She made sure that if the opportunity arose I wouldn't miss out, by telling all the other staff. I really appreciated this compared to other placements where I received such a negative experience from people whom I asked for help.

Reflective activity

Compare two areas where you have had very differing levels of clinical practice facilitation and identify what you did differently in those practice areas.

Experience is gained through seeing how others do things, or what happens in a particular context; however, if someone is new to a situation, they may not know what to look for, and it can be very easy to miss opportunities and to notice very little. This problem can be reduced by the use of a simple observation checklist that covers what to look out for and perhaps asks the learner to record events and how often they happened. Simple checklists can be devised by the learner or with the assistance of the mentor/supervisor. For example, prior to seeing a physiotherapist mobilizing a patient for the first time following hip replacement surgery, the physiotherapist and the student or students could have a short discussion about what to look out for, and devise a brief checklist. Afterwards, the list could be used to structure a short discussion which encourages reflection on what has been seen and the significance that these observations have for future practice.

It can be difficult to undertake a task effectively if you do not have a sound understanding of what would count as doing it well. It makes an enormous difference to how attentive a learner is when undertaking a practical task if they have a clear idea of the criteria that will be used to judge the outcome of their work.

Many higher education institutes have developed their own student's charter which gives guidance about the learner's rights and responsibilities in relation to clinical practice. These are often written with involvement from placement providers as well as the health care teaching staff. If a student charter is available, both the mentor and student should be aware of its content.

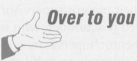

Over to you

Find out if your locality has a student charter, and take a look at its content. Ask yourself if all of these standards are being met.

Conduct on placement

A health care student becomes closely involved with the public in a professional capacity and, therefore, should at all times work in a manner acceptable to the profession to which they aspire and follow the guidance on professional conduct. The NMC have published 'Your guide to practice' (2011b) which sets out the personal and professional conduct expected of student nurses and student midwives. When on placement, the learner has access to confidential and personal information relating to patients/clients and sensitive information relating to other members of staff who are work colleagues. It is important to remember to maintain confidentiality even outside the clinical environment.

Reflective activity

Whilst travelling home on the bus from an early shift, you hear a member of staff discussing a patient whom they are treating. Although you do not know this health carer, you can identify the area/placement in which they work and the patient details being discussed are fairly specific. Think about what you could/might do.

- Have you ever experienced a situation where a student or colleague was not professional in their conduct, and how did this make you feel?
- How did you deal with the situation?

Whatever the dress code for the clinical area, the learner has a responsibility to adhere to this, promoting a professional image and keeping to health and safety policies. An identification badge should be worn at all times in clinical areas.

Different placement areas may vary in their working patterns and shifts, and the student should be made aware of these details prior to commencing the placement. The student will be expected to adopt the placement's duty rotas, which may include working early and late shifts, weekends, and night duty where this is the normal pattern of working. In many placements, the student is supernumerary and, therefore, takes on the same duty rota as their mentor or supervisor; however, adjustment may be made to ensure that the student has experience in all aspects of care within the speciality or to take account of the student's personal commitments. If a student is not working with their mentor/supervisor because of sickness or a differing shift pattern, the registered practitioner, who is responsible for that particular shift, acts as the associate mentor/supervisor.

All attendance on a placement should be recorded accurately to fulfil the requirements of the health care programme; there may be a specified number of clinical hours to be achieved by the end of a professional course. If the student is unable to attend a clinical placement as scheduled, they must inform the clinical staff prior to the start of the shift. Usually, in addition, the higher education institute also needs to be informed of any sickness or absence. The student should also inform the placement area and the higher education institute of their return from sickness or absence.

Students should keep themselves informed regarding placement allocations and any changes and should prepare for the impending speciality.

Clinical staff can provide mentorship, supervise the student's experience and assess their practice according to the requirements of their course. Health professionals, other than nurses and midwives and other members of staff, all contribute to your learning experiences, so make sure that you engage with the multidisciplinary team. In a small case study exploring reasons why nursing students consider leaving their course Bowden (2008) found that the stress of undertaking clinical placements was the second most common reason cited.

CHANGING CURRICULA

In nursing, there has been a movement away from what was broadly apprenticeship training with education delivered in NHS nursing departments to pre-registration programmes of education delivered within higher education institutes (HEIs) and leading to a minimum academic qualification at diploma level. There has also been increased access to post-registration qualifications at degree and higher degree levels.

Sometimes, an 'unfortunate split' between cognitive and practical skills has inadvertently been reinforced by a curriculum development team, with 'practical skills being relegated to a position of 'secondary importance' (Elkan and Robinson, 1993). Decontextualized skills learnt in the university are not transferable to the workplace, and the fragmented, information-driven view of professional knowledge leads to a piecemeal collection of knowledge without an understanding of how it fits together (Bechtel *et al.*, 1999; Richardson, 1999). Edmond (2001) suggests that education for all practice disciplines is undergoing a paradigm shift, where the value of practical education and experience will be better understood and integrated with theoretical knowledge. This cultural shift has required a movement away from 'clinical education by default', reduced emphasis on front-loading theory, and increased structure for practical experiences (Eraut *et al.*, 1998).

Looking back on curricula changes within nursing, it is clear that a radical educational shift occurred with the implementation of 'Project 2000' pre-registration curricula. The major aim of Project 2000 curricula was to deliver knowledgeable nurses for the future. In 1999, the Department of Health and the United Kingdom Central Council for Nursing, Midwifery and Health Visiting (UKCC) recommended the strengthening of education and training for nurses (UKCC/DoH, 1999). The 'fitness for practice' model called for increased flexibility within curricula, partnership working between HEIs and NHS Trusts, and initiatives to ensure that students were able to meet the future roles envisaged for registered nurses (DoH, 2000b).

Main changes in 'fitness for practice' curriculum

- Increased student intakes to meet NHS requirements which required additional practice placements.
- Flexible approaches to access and accreditation of prior (experiential) learning (APEL).
- Earlier allocations of students to practical placements from the start of their course.
- An identified 'base ward' to increase 'ownership' of the students by the service providers.
- Improved integration of theory and practice throughout the course, with an emphasis on clinical practice and the development of transferable critical appraisal skills.

- Strengthened partnership links between higher education institutes and NHS Trusts.

- A shorter common foundation programme (reduced from 18 months to one year).

- Wider assessment of practice skills by practice supervisors (mentors) through the development of practice evidence.

- A need to demonstrate competence at the end of pre-registration education with a period of preceptorship following registration.

Learning-centred curricula identify learning outcomes reflecting current nursing practice and the user's perspective (Bailey, 2005) and use authentic assessment to evidence these (Candela *et al.*, 2006). Problem-based learning involves the simultaneous addressing of skills, knowledge and professional attitudes through group work and experiential learning which may transfer more easily to the clinical context.

KEY POINTS

Teaching methods that support the integration of theory and practice are:

- Problem-based learning (can be based around one patient case, a patient problem, a clinical skill, an ethical or professional dilemma)

- Team teaching involving lecturers and clinical staff

- Accrediting work-based learning

- Recording and reviewing role-play communications

- Well-designed interactive e-learning with sufficient computer access time and skills (Atack and Rankin, 2002)

- Access to evidence-based information within academic and practical settings

- Clinical skills laboratories that allow the simulation of health care environments

- Action learning sets

- Patient teaching

- Tutorials and discussion groups

- Workshops

- Personal development plans

EVIDENCE BASE

The involvement of patients in teaching health care professionals has most successfully been integrated into mental health and learning disabilities curricula. Take a look at the following two articles:

● McGarry, J. and Thorn, N. (2004) How users and carers view their involvement in nurse education. *Nursing Times*, **100**(18), 36–39.

● Towle, A., Bainbridge, L., Godolphin, W., Katz, A., Kline, C., Lown, B., Madularu, I., Solomon, P. and Thistlewaite, J. (2010) Active patient involvement in the education of health professionals. *Medical Education*, **44**(1): 56–74.

Health professional education has undergone a number of changes over the past 20 years, reflecting national educational trends and service changes. For example, nursing practice is changing, with nurses in acute settings caring for increasingly complex patient problems and acutely sicker patients with co-morbidities within a demographic population change where there are more older people; and nurses in community and primary care settings working with raised levels of patients living with long term conditions and needing to encourage self-care wherever possible (RCN, 2004). This trend is leading to a shift from hospital-based care to community-based care (Wanless, 2004). These service changes create challenges for curricular planning, which needs to offer increased student participation in community-based experiences (Gaines *et al.*, 2005).

Health care curricula are now required to integrate interprofessional learning to prepare staff adequately for their future work roles. A definition of interprofessional education can be 'occasions when two or more professions learn with, from and about each other to improve collaboration and quality of care (CAIPE, 2002). Interprofessional education incorporates the arrangements made for people from different disciplines and professions to learn with each other, and it has been suggested that the term 'interprofessional' implies that professions should learn from and about each other to improve collaboration, rather than just learn side by side. Advocates of interprofessional learning perceive that it promotes teamwork and cultivates collaborative practice. Interprofessional education involves the application of the principles of interactive adult learning (discussed in Chapter 2) to interprofessional group-based learning (Wigens, 1999). There are many instances reported of the successful outcomes from interprofessional education experiences, and students tend to value these most when assessment of this is integral to their health care programme (Barr *et al.*, 2011).

Reflective activity

Think about when you have participated in interprofessional learning. What was the subject area? (Common areas for interprofessional learning often include communication, documentation, problem solving, critical thinking, management, research, ethics, reflective practice and clinical supervision.) In your opinion, was the topic an appropriate area for interprofessional learning and was it handled well, so that all participants' contributions were valued?

Opportunities for nurses and other health care professionals to learn together should be taken: not just by getting professionals into the classroom together but by sharing learning through meaningful projects. Being critically aware of the influence of context (or presage factors) can inform interprofessional education decisions (Freeth and Reeves, 2004). There are logistical difficulties in organizing interprofessional educational curricula, and a clinical hierarchy can affect interprofessional working, with some members being perceived as having more professional knowledge and status (Pirrie *et al.*, 1998). Placing professionals together in multidisciplinary groups does not necessarily guarantee the development of a shared understanding. For instance, student nurses who shared lectures with medical and allied health professional students in their first year did not appear to develop an enthusiastic approach to multidisciplinary working (Pirrie *et al.*, 1998). Student nurses often sat in segregated groups, and they expressed concerns about the lack of opportunities to consolidate their own sense of professional identity before introducing interprofessional education within their programme (Pirrie *et al.*, 1998).

Evidence as to the effectiveness of interprofessional education from the first systematic reviews indicates that interprofessional education is happening in a wide range of health care programmes at pre- and post-qualification levels (Barr *et al.*, 2011). Positive changes in knowledge and skills have been found, and some evidence shows that interprofessional learning has an impact on patient outcomes (Barr *et al.*, 2011; Hammick, 2000). It is suggested that health care professionals should be educated to function as team members, which would be helped by a consensus about the competencies that graduates should achieve (Stephenson *et al.*, 2002).

Parity in educational curricula has become important, and the RCN (2004) suggested that the transition to an all graduate nursing profession had a certain inevitability, as most health care professions have their initial qualifications linked to gaining a degree. There has been, however, scepticism about advocating an all-graduate nursing workforce Miers (2002) suggests that there is anti-intellectualism within nursing which has been fuelled by those in practice who critique nursing academia. This view is supported by the suggestion that there has been a denigration of practice by those who are solely based within nursing institutes of higher education, with these nursing academics valuing propositional knowledge over other forms of knowledge. Heitlinger (1999) suggests that the movement of nursing education into higher education has benefited nurses, as the location of their education within universities has increased their political position in comparison with other health care professionals. Those advocating a degree-level pre-registration qualification argue that theoretical learning does not preclude practical ability (RCN, 2004).

Nursing students currently complete their education with at least a Diploma in Higher Education – the equivalent of two thirds of a degree. This has served well for more than 10 years, with nurses largely being seen as well prepared to meet current service needs when they qualify.

The NMC (2010b) published new Standards for pre-registration education which reflect how future services are likely to be delivered, acknowledge future public health priorities and address the challenges of long-term conditions, an ageing population, and providing more care outside hospitals. Nurses must be equipped to lead, delegate, supervise and challenge other nurses and health care professionals. They must be able to develop practice, and promote and sustain change.

Professional values must underpin education as well as practice. All students are obliged to adhere to guidance on professional conduct for nursing and midwifery students (NMC, 2011b), the code is central to all education programmes, and educators must enable students to understand, commit to and uphold it.

It is argued that the challenges for nursing in the 21st century are much more complex and health care delivery is changing. New education programmes will aim to ensure that nurses, when they graduate in their field of practice, will have the high level skills needed to care for people in their particular field, while also having the knowledge and range of skills needed to provide essential care to anyone else in any setting. In order to complete their education programmes successfully, nursing students will have to demonstrate knowledge and competence in practice at degree level. This means that they have to be able to justify their actions based on evidence. The NMC believes that degree-level nurses will be able to provide a better standard of care. Degree level pre-registration nursing programmes offered in the UK ensure that the nursing workforce is more independent and innovative, able to assess and apply effective evidence-based care, work in a multi-disciplinary environment and across service boundaries providing leadership: promoting, sustaining change and the development of clinical services (NMC, 2010b).

Nurse educational programmes are particularly appreciated if they assess 'learning in practice' by allowing individuals to immerse themselves in practice (Wigens, 2004). Immersion in practice early on in a nursing career is seen as the way to learn nursing. Qualified staff view students as needing a lengthy time in practice, greater than four weeks, and believe that supernumerary status when fully realized has benefits (Wigens, 2004). However, the support for student nurses has to be balanced against the priority of care giving, and, therefore, support should be spread across the trained staff in the nursing team (Wigens, 2004). Learner support and confirmation of progress is not just the mentor's role but is seen as the role of the whole community of practice (Ohrling and Hallberg, 2001b; Phillips *et al.*, 2000a; Wigens, 2004). Individual learning becomes community learning through the process of disseminating and discussing individual knowledge within a team. Student nurses relate to a learning environment by their perception of the quality of nursing care and patient relationships (Papastavrou *et al.*, 2010).

EVIDENCE BASE

Read: Papastavrou, E., Lambrinou, E., Tsangari, H., Saarikoski, M. and Leino–Kilpi, H. (2010) Student nurses experience of learning in the clinical environment. *Nurse Education Practice*, **10**(3): 176–182.

   This research was undertaken in Cyprus. What is your view of the likelihood of the same findings being found in your country?

Nurse education courses should look at current and future nursing practice and be assessed through work-based routes, such as portfolios of practice evidence. Classroom activities grounded in everyday situations recognize that knowledge is acquired in the situation and involves the social processes of thinking, perceiving and problem solving. Wenger (1998) suggests that the curriculum should be an itinerary of transformative experiences, maximizing interactions – rather than just a list of subject matter. Using problem-based learning, reflecting on incidents and discussing the knowledge underpinning practice is more likely to be a transformative experience having longer-term significance than extensive coverage of broad, abstract and general curricula.

MECHANISMS TO ENSURE PLACEMENTS ARE EFFECTIVE

Clinical placements are considered to be the most influential aspects of nurse education programmes and this is likely to be the case for many health care programmes. The NMC has said that the most recently published 'Standards for pre-registration education' (2010b, p. 4)

" *.. aim to enable nurses to give and support high quality care in rapidly changing environments. They reflect how future services are likely to be delivered, acknowledge future public health priorities and address the challenges of long-term conditions, an ageing population, and providing more care outside hospitals. Nurses must be equipped to lead, delegate, supervise and challenge other nurses and health care professionals. They must be able to develop practice, and promote* *and sustain change. As graduates they must be able to think analytically, use problem-solving approaches and evidence in decision-making, keep up with technical advances and meet future expectations.*

Care in clinical placements needs to be evidence-based and reflect respect for the rights of service users, including maintaining their dignity, privacy and religious needs. Students are exposed to a variety of care approaches, as each placement will have its own philosophy and model of care in use. However, every placement should adhere to all relevant local and governmental policies and procedures.

Placements must be effectively prepared for student allocation and should provide an equitable opportunity for each individual to achieve their respective placement outcomes. Institutions should ensure that students are provided with appropriate guidance and support in preparation for, during and after their placements; this includes:

- appropriate induction to the placement environment including health and safety information
- any occupational health, legal or ethical considerations or requirements (e.g. patient confidentiality)
- the means of recording the achievement of learning outcomes
- availability of additional skills preparation
- cultural orientation and work expectations
- institutional support services that students can access.

Students should be given an opportunity to evaluate a placement so that the clinical staff, managers and the higher education institute can work on the areas for improvement or celebrate and disseminate 'good practice'. This usually takes the form of a questionnaire, but is also strengthened by a discussion at the end of the placement period. The questionnaire usually focuses on the welcome received, the range of clinical experience gained, opportunities provided to communicate with staff and patients, whether the placement allowed achievement of the learning outcomes, the level of feedback and support from mentors/supervisors, and the availability and access to resources. These resources can be in the form of journals, other publications, the Internet, multidisciplinary forums, specialist 'spoke' placements and the physical space for the student and mentor to meet. The benefit of using a questionnaire, in addition to verbal feedback, is aided if the questionnaire is completed anonymously. Some higher education institutes add some free-text boxes for detailed comments on strengths and areas for improvement.

What universities need to ensure and monitor is the quality of the practice learning environment so that students experience a high quality learning and teaching experience which fosters their professional development and competence (Chan, 2002). Students who undertake nursing and midwifery programmes identify closely with practice as this is the reality of their chosen course of study. Students learn the culture and socialization of nursing and midwifery through practice experiences and therefore it is a fundamental, underpinning component of the pre-registration provision. Unlike the university experience, no practice placement is the same and this in itself can make it a challenge to evaluate the quality, effectiveness, and outcomes of these differing learning environments (Chan, 2002; Boor *et al.*, 2007; Bloomfield and Subramaniam, 2008).

Therefore the evaluation of practice placements by pre-registration students continues to be of a high priority. This feedback is utilized by the HEI to fulfil part of Quality Assurance mechanisms and NMC requirements, and acts as a guide for future planning, giving vital insight into the students' practice learning experience. This same information can also be assimilated by the placement providers to construct a picture of the nature of the learning climate that they offer and enable the ongoing development of individual environments.

Many schools of nursing report that getting busy clinical staff and students to complete an evaluation tool is a perennial problem (Moseley *et al.*, 2004), so having an effective and simple tool is essential. Attempts to improve the placement evaluation have been made (RCN, 2002a), and Moseley *et al.* (2004) have empirically tested their 15-statement tool (see Table 10.1 below) in the UK, Finland and Germany. A numerical rating can be placed alongside these statements allowing the generation of computerized reports, and individual and cohort tracking.

Table 10.1   Example of an evaluation of clinical placement questionnaire
1 During my first day/shift I was provided with a planned introduction to the practice placement area.
2 During my first day/shift I was allocated a supervisor/supervisory team.
3 A range of resources was available for my use in the placement area.
4 During my placement, the staff encouraged me to ask questions about practice/theory.
5 During my placement, staff used placement learning/teaching opportunities, which supported my learning needs.
6 During my placement, staff encouraged and supported me to learn as and when the opportunities arose.
7 During my first day/shift, I was given the name of my mentor/supervisor.
8 In the first part of my placement, my mentor/supervisor and I discussed how I could achieve the required skills and learning outcomes for the placement.
9 My mentor/supervisor and I set target dates and reviewed my progress as required by my course and as appropriate to my length of placement.
10 During the placement, I received feedback on my progress and discussed this with my mentor/supervisor.

(Continued)

Table 10.1   Example of an evaluation of clinical placement questionnaire (*Continued*)
11 On completion of my placement, all relevant documentation was completed, signed and dated by my mentor/supervisor as required by my course (e.g. learning contract, skills book, portfolio).
12 During each shift I was supervised by either a named mentor/supervisor or a small supervisory team.
13 I was able to discuss my level of supervision with my mentor/supervisor.
14 At all times during the placement I knew who was supervising me.
15 Placement details were made available to me at least two weeks before the placement start date.

Over to you

Take a look at the 15 statements included in the final evaluation tool (Table 10.1 above). Note that some of the wording (identified in italics) has been adapted.

- I got on well with the clinical staff.
- I had a good working relationship with the *mentor*/preceptor.
- Questions were answered satisfactorily.
- Staff explained procedures to me.
- I was treated as part of the team.
- The *mentor*/preceptor had a good sense of humour.
- Staff encouraged me to ask questions.
- The *mentor*/preceptor pointed out learning opportunities.
- Nurses gave me information about the care that they were giving to patients.
- The *mentor*/preceptor encouraged students to ask questions.
- The *mentor*/preceptor attached great importance to my learning needs.
- The more I put into the placement, the more I got out.
- I was motivated and keen to learn.
- Patients were well cared for.
- The *mentor*/preceptor was confident in their ability to teach me.

Compare the type of evaluative data that you would submit about your current placement/work area, using this tool with the data that would be elicited by the questionnaire example given previously.

As well as the evaluation of the placement, there should also be a structured debriefing session after the placement so that students within a cohort gain maximum benefit from their placement experiences. Debriefing activities can take many forms including group discussion, patient/user involvement, presentations, and drama workshops. The key facet of this debriefing is that students can discuss and share their experiences, clarify and present their learning and identify areas for further knowledge development. Wherever possible, practice-based learning should dovetail with classroom-based learning. We will explore how evaluation processes can be developed in the online bonus material accompanying this chapter.

ACADEMIC AND SERVICE PARTNERSHIPS

The current climate rewards universities and the NHS working together. Whilst the mentor retains accountability and responsibility for their student they are only part of the context: the clinical leader; clinical and learning environment; the Higher Education Institution; and service provided by the placement all contribute to the experience. Collaboration requires a closer partnership between lecturers, the HEI and the employers and services involved. However, having different 'communities of nurse academics' and 'communities of practitioners' means that these have distinct cultures (Mulhall, 2002). Practitioners consider that much of the research generated by academics asks irrelevant questions, lacks generalization and has unrealistic resource implications (Mulhall, 2002), but academic–service partnerships that support the development of evidence-based practice are viewed as a fruitful area for collaboration. A research and evidence-based practice ethos needs to be championed at varying levels within organizations with forums for dissemination, such as specialist nurse link groups.

EVIDENCE BASE

Take a look at Perry-Woodford, Z. and Whayman, K. (2005) Education in practice: a colorectal link-nurse programme. *British Journal of Nursing*, **14**(16): 862–866.

This article suggests that link nurses, who attend an education programme and are given time to undertake this role, have an increased awareness of the overall patient pathway and the role of the multidisciplinary team.

The implementation of research is strongly affected by clinical teams, requires 'old-timer' support, and needs to be applicable to the resource-constrained setting (Wigens, 2004). Nursing communities of practice find their own ways of connecting evidence-based knowledge to their everyday knowledge to achieve change. Nurses often read research evidence when they have access to it through CPD activities, as Thompson *et al.* (2001) found. Nurses also used oral story-telling about poor practice in the past as a way of showing allegiance to evidence-based practice (Burke and Smith, 2000). Education courses or conferences may be the catalyst for a care change as they provide access to evidence from outside the nursing team. Senior nurses talk of 'pushing' to put evidence-based changes in place, a process which involves a transformation of the evidence into a context-sensitive form (Greenhalgh and Worrall, 1997). Facilitators of change need to know the context to justify their actions to others. Frameworks for evidence-based practice require sufficient flexibility for community interpretation within practice settings and are best developed within teams, either interprofessional or nursing specific as appropriate. Crucial to a 'learning culture' is the range of opportunities for discussion and debate about nursing practice.

Trust-wide frameworks can help embed evidence-based practice changes. A clinical guideline, for instance, can help a clinical team but the technical knowledge contained within a guideline still requires interpretation and has to be flexible enough 'in action' to be applicable to different clinical settings. There is less scepticism concerning guidelines and the possibility of these reducing professional practice (Stevens and Ledbetter, 2000) than might be expected, so long as guidelines are sufficiently flexible to fit into their 'real-world' setting (Eraut, 2000b). Opportunities for staff to see an evidence-based practice change working in another clinical area, or being used by a practitioner in their own clinical area, strengthen the chance of this change being adopted throughout a clinical setting. Using ideas and ways of working from other contexts can have a powerful impact on transforming practice.

As well as the academic–service partnerships created through evidence-based practice, the need for effective support of learners is also displayed when both the HEI and the placement provider are evaluated and quality assured in partnership in relation to health care educational programmes. Placement providers need to be open and transparent about any concerns regarding the quality of care or staffing issues in a placement which are negatively affecting patient and student experience. Any regulatory concerns should be shared with the HEI team, e.g. Care Quality Commission initial feedback following an unannounced inspection visit. The 'partners' included health professional councils, the Department of Health, Commissioning groups, NHS Trusts, and HEIs need to work collaboratively together to get the best learning environments. This will support:

1 benchmarking and quality standards
2 programme approval
3 ongoing quality monitoring and enhancement
4 reviews
5 development of a shared evidence base on which conclusions and judgements are based.

Self- and peer evaluation is undertaken, supported by evidence, to identify strengths and issues in relation to practice and campus learning, and action plans are proposed to improve the quality of education.

Practice placements and campus-based learning are both quality assured as they are seen as integral to the whole health professional educational programme. The way that educational programmes are now quality assured acknowledges service providers' explicit role as practice educators.

EDUCATIONAL ROLES

There are a number of educational roles that support learning within a health care organization. In previous chapters, you will have looked at the mentor, preceptor, practice teacher and clinical supervisor roles. In this section, we examine other educational roles.

Over to you

Find out what educational posts are within your locality – some examples are listed here. Try to find out how to contact any of the following:

- education and training leads (may be within a human resources, education or nursing department)
- link lecturers
- practice educators
- trainers, e.g. resuscitation, moving and handling
- clinical practice facilitators
- practice education facilitators
- professional development nurses
- work-based learning/NVQ co-ordinators.

Ask at least two people in these roles what they consider to be their main aims within their current position.

Situated learning in practice can be fostered by educational roles; within this section these roles are broadly discussed under the title 'practice educator'. There are two models for practice educator implementation:

- the practice educator is based within the nursing/clinical team
- the practice educator visits a range of clinical areas.

If educational roles are sited within communities of practice, rather than educational facilitation being a visiting, auxiliary function, practice educators are more likely to play an integral part in the developing of personal development plans for staff members and formalized support structures. This can, however, be a costly model for practice education within an organization, and visiting educational roles are, therefore, often used to enhance learning.

It is essential that practitioners are self-directed, but they must also appreciate the role of others as catalysts for their learning. Practice educators can act as critical companions helping practitioners to develop expertise, as they act as a resource and provide high levels of challenge and support (Manley *et al.*, 2005). External influences on the nursing teams are limited, so the role of these 'brokers' within communities of practice is important (Wenger, 1998). Brokers have multi-membership of communities of practice, and they help the transfer of practice from one community to another. They help create connections, but there is a fine balance between being seen as full members of one community and being rejected as an intruder in another. External facilitation by practice educators can allow staff to review the importance of the shared values that underpin current practice, without dictating a particular change in practice.

Human sources (clinically trusted and credible individuals) are overwhelmingly perceived as the most useful in reducing the uncertainties of nursing decisions (Thompson *et al.*, 2001). Clinical credibility is a necessary condition for perceiving a source of evidence, such as a practice educator, as useful. However, even though guidance is derived from others, one cannot assume that this has no basis in research knowledge.

A practice educator was asked about their role. Their responses have been summarized below.

Health care professional

Practice educator

The advert for the Practice Development Nurse role was attractive to me because other institutions often want the person to be a full-time manager and full-time practitioner, as well as taking on this role. Senior staff try to take on this role, although they do not have the title, and the PDN role formalizes this responsibility.

I saw my key objective was to 'Risk manage education within the department', as there is a need to 'fit in' the education developments and identified education needs, requiring a commitment to prioritize covering staff time to access courses.

I make sure that I am visible on the 'shop floor'. If someone is off sick the staff are encouraged to try and seek a replacement, rather than to assume that the PDN will fill in, but if there is a crisis I will work with a member of staff in a mentoring role. When working with staff there is questioning and coaching regarding practice as the care is delivered.

When there are vacancies, especially at a senior level within a department/ward, there can be a constant battle between the PDN role and function and service needs. This can cause a 'guilty conscience' that you cannot stop – it is always there, although the PDN needs to maintain clinical credibility. I meet up with two other PDNs to receive group clinical supervision, and balancing the need to facilitate learning and cover care delivery are constantly coming up as an issue.

The team days I arrange are not viewed as 'optional' and good rostering is the key. To encourage people to attend, there need to be visible benefits (e.g. development of Patient Group Directives). Study days are easier to plan for, as you cannot take people out for an hour at a time as this affects the service. The PDN needs to ensure that they do not de-skill those interested in the facilitation of learning. For instance, one of the staff continues to co-ordinate the mentorship of student nurses, whilst the PDN in this case focuses on registered staff and support staff.

The practice educator talking in the last excerpt had a dedicated educational role. Field (2004) has suggested that practice educators may be clinically and academically competent, but that their lack of constant clinical engagement can mean that they have less clinical expertise when compared with mentors and clinical supervisors. A learning organization is likely to invest in dedicated educational roles as well as in those who integrate support of practice-based learning with a defined clinical workload.

Nurse teachers, too, have a role in supporting learning in practice. The NMC states that 20 per cent of the normal teaching hours of nurse teachers should be taken up with supporting learning in practice (NMC, 2008). This can be done in many ways.

Nurse teacher activities to support learning through practice

- Acting as a link lecturer
- Supporting mentor and practice teacher development
- Active clinical role
- Professional and practice development
- Contributing to practice research
- Involvement in action learning sets
- Supporting clinical leadership development

Finding an appropriate role for the nurse teacher within practice, as well as higher education, has created some difficulties. The role of the nurse teacher has been perceived in the past as becoming more 'academic' and less committed to nursing practice (Crotty, 1993), and some students have become dissatisfied with the type and frequency of their interactions with the nurse teachers. There is a need for clarification of the current confusion regarding the clinical role of nurse lecturers and for nurse lecturers to have an active presence in practice settings, maintaining their clinical knowledge and credibility (Ioannides, 1999). Educational activities can only be directly related to practice if nurse lecturers have a strong working relationship with clinical practice. If nurse educators are to function as facilitators of learning, they need to identify their role within practice or they will be unable to show authenticity in their subject matter (Wigens, 2004). Nurse teachers can facilitate practice-based learning, and practice educator roles can also cross over into higher education with mutual benefit.

The NMC teacher standard, which applies to practice educators and nurse teachers who support learning in practice and academic environments, requires them to have at least three years' post-registration experience on the same part of the professional register as the learners they support. They should hold a first degree and an approved teacher preparation post-graduate qualification (this is usually a year-long course which involves 360 hours assessed teaching) (NMC, 2008).

EVIDENCE BASE

The NMC postgraduate teacher qualification is also recognized by the Higher Education National Academy (HENA) which specifies that evidence of teaching activities, core/specialist knowledge and professional values are necessary to meet the national standard (HENA, 2006).

Take a look at the following website: **www.heacademy.ac.uk**

Practice educators require support, just like students and junior colleagues, but have a tendency to focus on meeting the needs of students and their mentors, neglecting their own professional support requirements. Nurses in senior roles who are helping to support learning through practice may be quite isolated and may find that educational and professional support mechanisms are lacking. A new nurse teacher often has an identified mentor who is an experienced educator. However, as time progresses there is often no formalized support role identified and it is tacitly expected that teachers will develop their own educational support network, outside the usual academic line management. Stress levels can be high within education, with the general pressures of academic life being compounded by schemes to assess the quality of teaching and research (Ioannides, 1999). A nurse lecturer can benefit from an identified clinical colleague who acts as a clinical support to the lecturer.

Peer clinical supervision may be in place for practice educators; however, this can be reduced by the everyday fluctuations in supervisory and teaching workloads. Cushen and Wigens (2000) advocate the setting up of transformational partnerships between lecturers, practice educators and senior clinical nurses, whereby nurses working in different organizations or specialities can provide mutual clinical support. This partnership can assist professional and personal development as well as giving time out to reflect on practice. A transformational partnership should be an equal relationship, where peers work together in a collegiate fashion, empowering partners to work to their full potential, by challenging current working and encouraging a sense of direction. There has to be respect and understanding of each other's unique perspective on learning through practice.

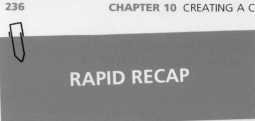

RAPID RECAP

Check your progress in learning from this book and from this last chapter in particular by working through each of the following questions.

1 Define the term 'reality shock' and identify the possible stages of this.

2 Give four teaching methods that could help to integrate theory and practice.

3 Why are academic and service partnerships being encouraged?

4 What reasons could a learning organization give for encouraging the continuous professional development of its employees?

5 What activities may a nurse teacher undertake within a clinical setting?

If you have difficulty with one of these questions, read through the section again to refresh your understanding.

APPENDIX

MAPPING TO NMC AND PRACTICE EDUCATOR STANDARDS

	NMC Standard to Support Learning and Assessment in Practice (2008, Section 2 – NMC standards for mentors, practice teachers and teachers, 2.1.2 Competence and outcomes for a mentor)	Common standards for: Chartered society of physiotherapy www.csp.org.uk **Accreditation of clinical educators (ACE)** College of Occupational Therapists www.cot.co.uk **Accreditation of practice placement educators (APPLE)** College of Radiographers www.sor.org **Practice Educator Accreditation scheme (PEAS)**
1 MENTORSHIP AND CLINICAL SUPERVISION SKILLS – AN INTRODUCTION * understand the overall structure and content of this book * start to understand the concept of learning through practice * recognize how this book has relevance to yourself as a learner and to your support of others in clinical settings * appreciate how important learning through practice is in bridging the theory and practice 'gap'.		
2 LEARNING FROM AND IN CLINICAL PRACTICE * Explain adult and higher education perspectives on learning * Appreciate the differences between behaviourist, cognitive and humanistic theories of learning * Understand the importance of lifelong learning and continuous professional development to professional practice * Understand your increasing involvement as a team member in the clinical environment * Anticipate the challenges of entering different communities of practice and how this impacts on your professional identity.	*Establishing working relationships* *Facilitation of learning* *Assessment and accountability* *Evaluation of learning* *Create an environment for learning* *Evidence based practice* *Leadership*	Apply learning theories that are appropriate for adult and professional learners Plan, implement and facilitate learning in the clinical setting Evaluate the learning experience Reflect on experience and formulate action plans to improve future practice
3 MENTORSHIP IN NURSING AND MIDWIFERY * Identify the roles that support learners within practice * Recognize the expectations of your professional body * Appreciate the common challenges encountered by all health care professionals when supporting learning in practice * Develop an awareness of the strategies to support an underachieving learner.	*Facilitation of learning* *Assessment and accountability* *Evaluation of learning* *Create an environment for learning* *Evidence-based practice* *Leadership*	Describe the role and identify the attributes of the effective clinical educator Apply sound principles and judgement in the assessment of performance in the clinical setting

(Continued)

4 MODELS OF PROFESSIONAL DEVELOPMENT AND SUPPORT – PRECEPTORSHIP AND CLINICAL SUPERVISION

* Define the main facilitator roles that support the learning of registered practitioners within practice
* Appreciate the importance of preceptorship and clinical supervision
* Explore methods of enhancing clinical skills development and assessment
* Value interpersonal communication and relationship building in allowing the effective giving and receiving of feedback.

Establishing working relationships
Assessment and accountability
Evaluation of learning
Create an environment for learning
Context of practice
Evidence based practice
Leadership

Describe the role and identify the attributes of the effective clinical educator
Apply learning theories that are appropriate for adult and professional learners
Plan, implement and facilitate learning in the clinical setting
Apply sound principles and judgement in the assessment of performance in the clinical setting
Reflect on experience and formulate action plans to improve future practice

5 IDENTIFYING INDIVIDUAL LEARNING NEEDS

* Explain the factors that affect your learning
* Undertake an assessment of your learning style
* Appreciate the need to balance individual learning needs with job/role requirements
* Discuss the structure and process of developing a learning contract or a personal development plan.

Establishing working relationships
Facilitation of learning
Assessment and accountability
Evaluation of learning
Leadership

Describe the role and identify the attributes of the effective clinical educator
Apply learning theories that are appropriate for adult and professional learners
Plan, implement and facilitate learning in the clinical setting

6 EXPERIENTIAL LEARNING AND THE ROLE OF REFLECTION

* Define the concepts of peer learning, problem-based learning and praxis
* Utilize reflective frameworks to review practice decision-making
* Explore team facilitation and action learning
* Value evidence-based practice and pragmatic approaches to action-planning.

Establishing working relationships
Facilitation of learning
Assessment and accountability
Evaluation of learning
Create an environment for learning
Evidence based practice

Describe the role and identify the attributes of the effective clinical educator
Apply learning theories that are appropriate for adult and professional learners
Plan, implement and facilitate learning in the clinical setting

7 FOCUSING ON ASSESSMENT

* Explain the main aspects of the assessment of practice
* Explore the concept of expertise and the journey from novice to expert

Establishing working relationships
Facilitation of learning
Assessment and accountability
Evaluation of learning

Apply sound principles and judgement in the assessment of performance in the clinical setting

(Continued)

* Understand skills teaching and the linkage with assessment criteria

Content	Standards	Outcomes
7 FOCUSING ON ASSESSMENT * Appreciate factors involved with setting your expectations in regard to assessment * Identify a range of evidence to utilize within practice.		
8 TECHNOLOGY IN 21st CENTURY PRACTICE, LEARNING AND TEACHING * Explain how using technology in education can enhance learning * Identify a range of technologies which are available * Appreciate the importance of remaining focused on the learning outcome * Start to identify opportunities for using technology in practice learning	*Facilitation of learning* *Assessment and accountability* *Evaluation of learning* *Create an environment for learning* *Leadership*	Plan, implement and facilitate learning in the clinical setting
9 INFLUENCES ON THE QUALITY OF PRACTICE LEARNING * Understand how issues, such as high patient caseloads and service improvement initiatives, can have an impact on learning through practice * Appreciate how multidisciplinary working can facilitate or hinder learning through practice * Acknowledge the role of emotional labour within health care * Recognize effective strategies to minimize the effect of constraints within varying contexts of practice.	*Establishing working relationships* *Facilitation of learning* *Assessment and accountability* *Evaluation of learning* *Create an environment for learning* *Context of practice* *Leadership*	Apply learning theories that are appropriate for adult and professional learners Evaluate the learning experience Reflect on experience and formulate action plans to improve future practice
10 CREATING A CLIMATE FOR LEARNING * Explain your professional code/guidelines for practice placements * Critically assess and evaluate a clinical area as a learning environment * Appreciate ways of getting the most from clinical environments; e.g. hub and spoke, teaching and learning programmes * Explain the main curricular changes that have occurred within health professional education	*Establishing working relationships* *Facilitation of learning* *Evaluation of learning* *Create an environment for learning* *Context of practice* *Evidence based practice* *Leadership*	

APPENDIX

RAPID RECAP ANSWERS

CHAPTER 1

1 What is situated learning?

Situated learning takes place in the setting where the learning will be applied, and assumes that social processes will affect this learning.

2 What is a community of practice?

A community of practice is where learning is seen as an act of membership and participation in a social group that integrates knowledge and situated learning into its life and working.

3 Define the term 'tacit knowledge'.

Tacit knowledge is rooted in context, people, places, ideas and experiences. A person carries tacit knowledge around in their mind from their experience; they may not consciously be aware of it, but it helps them to undertake their daily tasks.

4 Give some examples of evidence that could be used within a professional portfolio.

The range of evidence that can be offered to indicate learning through practice includes portfolios and profiles, reflective accounts, critical incident analyses, career biographies, learning diaries and competencies and skills documentation.

CHAPTER 2

1 What are the key differences between outcome-based and process-based learning?

The key differences between outcome- and process-based learning are that outcome-based learning is based on knowledge taken in and absorbed by the learner and retained for future use. It uses a building block approach, where knowledge is accumulated. Process-based learning involves a flexible network of ideas, knowledge and feelings, where learning involves a process of assembling, ordering or modifying understanding (termed assimilation by Piaget, 1971). Learning as a process is seen as grounded in experience, requiring a resolution of conflicts between alternative ways of looking at and adapting to the world. It involves transactions between the learner and the environment and leads to the creation of knowledge.

2 List the key principles underpinning:

(a) behaviourist theories of learning
(b) cognitive theories of learning
(c) humanistic theories of learning.

The key principles underpinning the following types of learning are:

- **Behaviourist** – from a behaviourist stance, learning is the result of the application of consequences, i.e. learners begin to connect certain responses with certain stimuli. There are two components to learning – Stimulus>Response. Different behavioural theories elaborate on this basic paradigm. Within the classical conditioning model, learning starts with an unconditioned response to an unconditioned (positive or negative) stimulus, a reflex. Other models focus on the consequences of the action, whether pleasant or otherwise. This adds another component to learning – Stimulus>Response>Outcome. An environmental event (for example a patient having a cardiac arrest) may act as a stimulus, and the outcome of the individual's response to the stimulus can be either negative or positive. Reinforcement will lead to a change in behaviour, either to increase or decrease the likelihood of the behaviour recurring.

- **Cognitive** learning is seen as coming from experience, reasoning and remembering information that allows the person to adapt to the environment. Learning involves the act of knowing, discovering and making meaning through intellectual processing and mental structuring. Understanding learning requires the study of information processing, as learning requires varying levels of elaboration moving from perception to the making of meaning. Remembering can be enhanced when, through experience, a person adds more connections to a single concept.

- **Humanistic** learning is focused on personal growth, the development of self-direction and interpersonal relationships. Behaviours are viewed as intentional and based on values, so to understand learning from this stance we need to study a person holistically as they grow and develop throughout their life. Feedback about learning is internal to the 'self' and based on individual motivations, goal setting and areas of interest.

3 **Explain the concepts 'lifelong learning' and 'continuous professional development'.**

Explanations of lifelong learning and continuing professional development are as follows:

- Lifelong learning has been defined as a process of accomplishing personal, social and professional development throughout the lifespan of the individual in order to enhance the quality of life of individuals and groups. It makes an assumption that learning takes place in all spheres of life, not just within educational institutes or in educational programmes.

- Continuous professional development is a range of learning activities through which professionals maintain and develop knowledge and expertise throughout their career to ensure that they retain their capacity to practise safely, effectively and legally within their evolving scope of practice.

4 **Why is it useful to be able to document learning through practice?**

It is useful to be able to document learning through practice because this can demonstrate to others a level of knowledge, competence or working. A student who is being assessed in relation to their practice learning will need to document their learning through practice to show how their theoretical and practical learning have become integrated. A qualified member of staff will document learning through practice evidence to demonstrate CPD achievement and a level of practice required to undertake their clinical role.

5 **Define the term 'hidden curriculum' within health care professional education.**

The 'hidden curriculum' within health care professional education means the unacknowledged, covert socializing processes of education that lead to the learning of cultural norms, values and beliefs.

6 **Explain in your own words what 'legitimate peripheral participation' means.**

Legitimate peripheral participation – this is where a student works within a community of practice, learning about the working of the clinical setting without full team membership

7 **Identify five factors that help the development of a community of practice clinical team.**

Factors that help the development of a community of practice clinical team are:

- Individuals learn and gain confidence by contributing to communities of practice.

- Communities are able to refine their practice whilst ensuring continued membership.

- The team transfer knowledge and skills throughout the membership.
- The clinical team can help staff invent and maintain ways of coping with the shifting 'real world' situation.
- The clinical team is able to use the process of legitimate peripheral participation to bring new members into the group whilst achieving continuity.
- Knowledge acquired in the authentic context has better chance of being activated when needed in another situation.
- Communities of practice are forums for situated knowledge and can assist in resolving conflict.

CHAPTER 3

1 What are the main responsibilities of a mentor:

- Identifying the needs of the learner
- Advising learners on the type of support available
- Providing guidance about facilities and learning resources in the organization
- Following up comments from other staff about students who are performing poorly or whose conduct is unacceptable
- Referring students with particular problems to the appropriate agencies
- Carrying out assessment of learning
- Completing the practice of assessment recording on completion of the placement

2 Which students require a sign off mentor?

Students on NMC approved pre-registration midwifery education programmes, leading to registration on the midwives' part of the register, can only be supported and assessed by mentors who have met the additional sign-off criteria. However students on pre-registration nursing programmes only require sign-off mentors on the final placement. Sign-off mentors are also required for all students on specialist practice programmes leading to a recordable qualification on the nurses' part of the register (NMC, 2008).

3 How should a mentor handle a situation where a student is performing poorly and is at risk of failing their practice assessment in the placement?

The mentor should meet with the student to discuss their progress and any concerns. They should seek the support of the HEI and seek the views of other mentors to share the responsibility and ensure fairness.

They need to state the problems clearly and listen to the student's views. An action plan should be developed identifying support requirements and expectation, deadlines for achievement should be set with review dates (all documented)

4 **What is a triennial review?**

The triennial review should provide evidence that mentors and practice teachers have mentored two students (one for practice teachers) in the last three years; and have participated in an annual update which included the opportunity to engage with other mentors. They should also have explored as a group the challenges to be encountered when assessing in challenging circumstances, and mapped their ongoing practice to the mentorship standards and ensured that they meet all these requirements to stay active on a 'live' register of mentors.

CHAPTER 4

1 **What are the main differences between mentorship and preceptorship?**

The main differences between mentorship and preceptorship are: A mentor:

- facilitates learning, supervises and assesses students during their clinical placements (usually around a 10–12 weeks' placement)
- is required to have successfully completed a Preparation for Mentorship qualification, usually at Level 3 (Hons degree) in order to undertake this role.

A preceptor:

- supports the growth and development of a novice registered practitioner
- fulfils this role for a fixed and limited amount of time with the specific purpose of assisting the novice into their new role (often four–six months)
- helps with the socializing of new team members into a practice community, helping them to become full members of the team.

2 **What issues need to be decided in order to formalize a preceptorship programme?**

In order to formalize a preceptorship programme, the following need to be agreed:

- the role of the preceptor, the relationship of the preceptor and preceptee within a preceptorship programme

- who requires preceptorship – for newly qualified staff, those returning from breaks in service and those returning after working for a significant time in a very different speciality
- the format for guidelines/documentation of the preceptorship period
- practical issues, training and support resources available, and how this differs from current arrangements

3 Define 'clinical supervision' and name two models/frameworks for clinical supervision.

Clinical supervision is a formal process with a skilled supervisor and supervisee. It should enable a professional to reflect on and assume responsibility for their practice, develop skills, knowledge and understanding of their practice whilst feeling supported. It is advocated for all clinical practitioners as it enhances consumer protection and safety of care in increasingly complex clinical situations.

Models/frameworks for clinical supervision are:

- Wagner's (1957) supervision triangle Heron's (1989) six-category intervention analysis
- Proctor's (1987) three-function interactive model
- Stoltenberg and Delworth's (1987) integrative development model

4 Why are ground rules necessary within clinical supervision?

Ground rules are necessary within clinical supervision to ensure that practitioners and supervisors are aware of what is involved and can trust in the confidentiality of clinical supervision.

CHAPTER 5

1 Identify a minimum of four factors that are likely to affect an individual's learning.

Four factors that are likely to affect an individual's learning are: motivation, personal life situation, employer support in providing either funding or study leave, and the learner's individual personality and learning style.

2 What is a reason for finding out someone's learning style? Give the names of two models that could be used to do this.

A reason for finding out someone's learning style is to enable them to become more motivated to learn by knowing more about their own strengths and weaknesses.

Models that could be used to do this are: the Dunn and Dunn Model; The Myers-Briggs Type Indicator (MBTI); Kolb's Learning Style Inventory (LSI) and Honey and Mumford's Learning Styles.

3 **What are the characteristics of information that can be used to help in the successful development of a learning objective?**

In order to develop a successful learning objective, ensure that the information you have should be SMART, i.e:

S P E C I F I C
M E A S U R A B L E
A C H I E V A B L E
R E A L I S T I C
T I M E B O U N D.

4 **What are the core dimensions of the NHS KSF and the role and responsibilities of an appraisee?**

The core dimensions of the NHS KSF are communication; personal and people development; health, safety and security; service improvement; development; quality; equality and diversity.

The role and responsibilities of an appraisee are to: understand the KSF outline for their post; evaluate their achievements referring to the KSF outline; identify their strengths; gather and structure evidence that demonstrates their achievements; identify their learning and development needs; prioritize, identify and arrange training and development activities to meet their learning needs; identify their personal contribution towards their personal development plan.

5 **Identify the five key components of a learning contract.**

The five key components of a learning contract or a personal development plan are:

● the knowledge, skills, attitudes, and values to be acquired by the learner (learning objectives)

● how these objectives are to be accomplished by the learner (learning resources and strategies)

● the target date(s) for completion

● what evidence will be presented to demonstrate that the objectives have been completed (evidence of accomplishment)

● how this evidence will be judged or validated (criteria and means for validating evidence) (Knowles, 1986).

CHAPTER 6

1 **How does experiential learning differ from classroom-based traditional teaching?**

Experiential learning differs from classroom-based traditional teaching as it encourages deep, rather than surface, approaches to learning. It is rooted in 'doing' and purposeful reflection, which gives meaning to experience and enables the discovery of knowledge that may not be evident through everyday experience alone.

2 List three frameworks that can guide reflection.

Three frameworks that can guide reflection are: Gibbs' reflective cycle structured reflection model; Palmer, Burns and Bulman's reflective framework; Johns' (2000) model of structured reflection.

3 What are the stages of the adapted Gibbs' reflective cycle?

The six stages of Gibbs' reflective cycle are: description, action plan, feelings, evaluation, conclusion and analysis.

4 What stages are there in making an evidence-based change in practice?

The stages in making an evidence-based change in practice are:

- Identify an area of practice.
- Undertake a literature review.
- Discuss the available literature with colleagues.
- Agree 'best practice' with colleagues.
- Compare 'best practice' to current practice.
- Make a change in practice if necessary.
- Evaluate the new practice.

5 Can you identify the components of a professional portfolio/profile?

A professional portfolio is a collection of individual material, providing proof of personal growth, continuing professional development, lifelong learning and competence. An effective portfolio is a visual representation of a practitioner's experience, strengths, abilities and skills. Cross-referencing, editing and imaginative paper management are important competencies in portfolio compilation. You need to split the evidence into logical sections, and if you are relating your evidence to a set of competences (Knowledge and Skills profile) it may be useful to use a cross-referencing grid or matrix.

CHAPTER 7

1 What are the key differences between:

(a) formative and summative assessment of practice

(b) criterion-referenced and norm-referenced assessment of practice?

(a)   The key differences between formative and summative assessment of practice are:

- Formative assessment takes place throughout the placement and is an informal assessment where the 'marks' do not count towards the final result. This type of assessment helps to identify strengths and weaknesses, and the level of student learning and progress. The assessor can use the formative assessment to identify a need for further explanation, additional practice experience, or whether learning can move on to other areas.

- Summative assessment usually takes place at the end of a placement and is a formal assessment where the 'mark' is used to determine the level of achievement. It can determine how much has been learnt by the student and the extent to which the learning outcomes have been met.

(b)   The key difference between criterion-referenced and norm-referenced assessment of practice is that criterion-referenced assessment relies on the explicit criteria provided by the education institute in order to make an assessment, whereas norm referencing compares students who are at the same stage of training and looks at how each is progressing compared with others in the group.

2 What are the level identifiers within Steinaker and Bell's (1979) experiential taxonomy?

The level identifiers within Steinaker and Bell's (1979) experiential taxonomy are:

- Exposure – the student has observed the skill being performed by a competent practitioner.
- Participation – the student has assisted a competent practitioner in the performance of the skill.
- Identification – the student has performed the skill under the supervision of a registered practitioner.
- Internalization – the student has sustained a skilled performance in a variety of settings under the supervision of a registered practitioner.
- Dissemination – the student has maintained professional competence and has enabled others to develop their knowledge and skills.

3 Identify at least six forms of evidence that could be included within a practice portfolio.

Forms of evidence that could be included within a practice portfolio are: observation of practical skills, student self assessment, discussion, learning contracts, guided study, written reflection, testimony of others, interviews, patient comments and feedback, peer evaluation, audit or data collection, case study, team project.

4 What methods can you use to assess practice?

Practice can be assessed by finding out what and how much a person has learnt, this can be through observation of practice, questioning knowledge and encompasses a range of methods to measure a learner's competence to practice clinical skills and gives an assessor an opportunity to provide feedback, support and guidance.

5 What should be done about patient information, when placing evidence that links patient care practice into an assessment-of-practice document?

When placing evidence that links to patient care practice into an assessment of practice document, patient information should be removed as patient confidentially should be maintained at all times.

CHAPTER 8

1 What is the difference between synchronous and asynchronous communication?

Synchronous communication occurs simultaneously and requires participants to engage in real time but not necessarily in the same place, whereas asynchronous communication is also free of the need to be in the same place but is not dependent on simultaneous exchanges.

2 List the key components of mobile learning.

Mobile learning provides the opportunity for anyone to access information and learning materials from anywhere and at any time through the use of wireless technology.

3 Explain how an e-portfolio can be used.

An e-portfolio can be used for a variety of different purposes including personal development, the presentation of work, or for assessment activities. They can cross organizational boundaries.

4 Describe what a virtual learning environment is.

The virtual learning environment is a 'learning platform' that is used as a repository for information, teaching and learning materials, submission of work for assessment and vehicle for giving feedback. Teaching and learning materials may include links to articles, podcasts, interactive quizzes, videos, links to webpages and so forth.

CHAPTER 9

1 What strategies may nurses use to cope with high workloads, time pressures and information overload?

The strategies that nurses may use to cope with high workloads, time pressures and information overload are:

- speeding up (acceleration)
- selecting the input of information (filtering)
- prioritizing
- using 'decision rules'
- omitting or avoiding
- locking on to one approach.

2 **What three phases do Crawford and Kiger (1998) suggest students progress through whilst on clinical placement?**

The three phases that Crawford and Kiger (1998) suggest that students progress through whilst on clinical placement are:

- adaptation (becoming part of the community)
- stabilization (increased knowledge and skills)
- consolidation (requiring reduced supervision.

3 **Outline the main aspects of the four models of practitioner–patient relationship.**

The main aspects of the four models of practitioner–patient relationship are:

(a) Nurse centred – This model influenced nursing in the past, and emphasized dependence of the patient on the health carer. Care giving was determined by the nurse who was viewed as more 'knowledgeable' than the patient. Care was delivered, it was perceived, in the patient's best interest.

(b) Technical relationship – Nursing is seen as a clinical science, where skilled, objective care is delivered without imposing any of the carer's values or wishes. In this model, the nurse's responsibility predominantly revolves around his or her technical competence. The patient may have the ultimate responsibility for determining needs, but the nurse informs and has current evidence and skills to impart.

(c) Patient centred – The nurse works alongside the patient, negotiating the role of the nurse as applicable to the situation and to individual patient needs. Within this model, there is the possibility for a therapeutic relationship to develop and for the nurse and patient to 'know' each other as people.

(d) Therapeutic relationship – Therapeutic relationship requires the nurse to respect and have genuine interest in the person, to show emotional warmth, tolerance and non-judgemental acceptance of the patient. It also calls for the practitioner to use 'self' in nursing interactions, whilst maintaining awareness of their limitations and adherence to ethical codes. The patient plays a part in a therapeutic relationship by trusting and co-operating with the intervention and being motivated to understand the treatment/care.

4 **What is meant by the term 'emotional labour'?**

The term emotional labour indicates the emotional work done as part of a job and is governed by 'feeling rules' set by the employer. These unarticulated rules of social interactions indicate how deeply we should feel and for how long. Expectations for emotional labour tend to be linked to female-dominated work roles.

5 **What do the letters PDSA stand for in the service improvement cycle?**

In the service improvement cycle, the letters PDSA stand for:
Plan / Do / Study / Act.

6 **How might a multidisciplinary team that could be described as 'committed' (Bruce, 1980) show that they are working interprofessionally?**

A multidisciplinary team described as 'committed' (Bruce, 1980) could show that they are working interprofessionally by investing time and energy into their teamwork.

CHAPTER 10

1 **Define the term 'reality shock' and identify the possible stages of this.**

'Reality shock' is the term used for conflict caused by, for example, the movement from the familiar higher education environment to the unfamiliar work setting, caused by a gap between what has been learnt and on-the-job experiences.

The possible stages of reality shock are:

- Honeymoon – the student is fascinated with the new work.
- Shock/rejection – the student rejects the new environment, or the old environment, or self and may become socially isolated.
- Recovery – the student is able to see the funny side of this, and is becoming competent.
- Resolution – the student is able to display culturally appropriate reactions.

2 **Give four teaching methods that could help to integrate theory and practice.**

Teaching methods that could help to integrate theory and practice are:

- problem-based learning (can be based around one patient case, a patient problem, a clinical skill, an ethical or professional dilemma)
- team teaching involving lecturers and clinical staff
- accrediting work-based learning
- recording and reviewing role-play communications
- well-designed interactive e-learning with sufficient computer access time and skills (Atack and Rankin, 2002)

- access to evidence-based information within academic and practical settings
- clinical skills laboratories that allow the simulation of health care environments
- action learning sets
- patient teaching
- tutorials and discussion groups
- workshops
- personal development plans.

3 **Why are academic and service partnerships being encouraged?**

Academic and service partnerships are being encouraged because they:

- enable sharing good practice and innovation nationally
- assist statutory bodies to maintain their obligations to protect the public
- provide evidence on the quality of higher education in health care provision
- ensure education is of a high quality for future employees.

4 **What reasons could a learning organization give for encouraging the continuous professional development of its employees?**

The reasons that a learning organization could give for encouraging the continuous professional development of its employees are:

- education and CPD activities impact on practitioners' ability to deliver health services as part of a flexible competent workforce (DoH, 1997).
- CPD enhances knowledge and skills
- there is a positive correlation between professional development and staff satisfaction, staff retention and quality patient care
- ability to access lifelong learning activities is aligned to recruitment and retention in the clinical setting.

5 **What activities may a nurse teacher undertake within a clinical setting?**

The activities that a nurse teacher may undertake within a clinical setting are:

- acting as a link lecturer, talking with staff and students
- supporting mentor and practice teacher development
- active clinical role
- professional and practice development
- contributing to practice research
- involvement in action learning sets
- supporting clinical leadership development.

REFERENCES

Abraham-Maslow (2012) Father of modern management [Online] available at http://www.abraham-maslow.com/m_motivation/Hierarchy_of_Needs.asp

Alderson, J. and Wall, D. (1993) Does washback exist? *Applied Linguistics*, **14**(2), 115–129.

Ali, P.A. and Panther, W. (2008) Professional development and the role of mentorship. *Nursing standard*, **22** (42) p. 35–39

Allan, H. T., Smith, P. and O'Driscoll, M. (2011) Experiences of supernumerary status and the hidden curriculum in nursing: a new twist in the theory-practice gap? *Journal of Clinical Nursing.* 20 p. 847–855

Allen, D. (2000) Negotiating the role of expert carers on an adult hospital ward. *Sociology of Health and Illness*, **22**(2), 149–171.

Ally, M. ed. (2009) *Mobile Learning Transforming the delivery of education and training* AU Press Edmonton AB.

Alzheimer's society (2012) 'This is me' [Online] available at http://alzheimers.org.uk/site/scripts/documents_info.php?documentID=1290

Andre, K. (2000) Grading student clinical practice performance: the Australian perspective. *Nurse Education Today*, **20**(8), 672–679.

Andrews, M. and Chilton, F. (2000) Student and mentor perceptions of mentor effectiveness. *Nurse Education Today*, **20**(7), 555–562.

Andrews, M. and Roberts, D. (2003) Supporting student nurses learning in and through practice: the role of the clinical guide. *Nurse Education Today*, **23**(7), 474–481.

Andrews, M., Brewer, M., Buchan, T., Denne, A., Hammond, J., Hardy, G., Jacobs, L., McKenzie, L. and West S. (2010) Implementation and sustainability of the Nursing and Midwifery Standards for Mentoring in the UK. *Nurse Education in Practice* **10**(5) 251–5

Armstrong, P. and Armstrong, H. (1996) *Wasting away. The undermining of Canadian health care.* Oxford University Press, Toronto.

Aston, L. and Hallam, P. (2011) *Successful Mentoring in Nursing.* Learning Matters. Exeter.

Atack, L. and Rankin, J. (2002) A descriptive study of registered nurses' experiences with web-based learning. *Journal of Advanced Nursing*, **40**(4), 457–465.

Audit Commission (2001) *Hidden Talents: education, training and development for health care staff in NHS Trusts.* Audit Commission National Report, London.

Bailey, D. (2005) Using an action research approach to involving service users in the assessment of professional competence. *European Journal of Social Work*, **8**(2), 165–179.

Banning, M. and Stafford, M. (2008) A hermeneutic phenomenological study of community nurses' CPD. *British Journal of Community Nursing.* **13**(4) p. 178–182

Barnett, R. (1997) *Higher Education: a critical business.* SRHE/Open University Press, Milton Keynes.

Barr, H., Hammick, M., Koppel, I. and Reeves, S. (1999) Evaluating interprofessional education: two systematic reviews for health and social care. *British Educational Research Journal*, **25**(4), 533–544.

Barr, H., Helm, M. and D'Avray, L. (2011) Developing Interprofessional Education in Health and Social Care Courses in the UK. A Progress Report: Occasional Paper 12. The Higher Education Academy: Health and Sciences Practice, London.

Barrett, H. (2002) Directions in Electronic Portfolio Development www.electronicportfolios.com

Batalden, P. and Stoltz, P. (1993) A framework for continuing improvement of health care: building and applying professional and improvement knowledge to test change in daily work. *The Joint Commission Journal on Quality Improvement*, **19**(10), 432–452.

Baxter Magolda, M. (1992) *Knowing and reasoning in college students: Gender-related patterns in students' intellectual development*. Jossey Bass, San Francisco

Bechtel, G., Davidhizar, R. and Bradshaw, M. (1999) Problem-based learning in a competency-based world. *Nurse Education Today*, 19(3), 182–187.

Bell, A., Horsfall, J. and Goodin, W. (1998) The mental health nursing clinical confidence scale: a tool for measuring undergraduate learning on mental health clinical placements. *Australian and New Zealand Journal of Mental Health*, 7(4), 184–190.

Benner, P. (1984) *From Novice to Expert: Excellence and power in clinical nursing practice*. Addison-Wesley, Menlo Park, California.

Biggs, J. (2003) *Teaching for Quality Learning at University*, 2nd edn. The Society for Research into Higher Education and Open University Press, Buckingham.

Bloomfield, L. and Subramaniam, R. (2008) Development of an instrument to measure the clinical learning environment in diagnostic radiology *Journal of Medical Imaging and Radiation Oncology* 52(3) p. 262–268

Bolton, S. (2001) Changing faces: nurses as emotional jugglers. *Sociology of Health and Illness*, 23(1), 85–100.

Boor, K., Scheele, F., Van der Vleuten, C.P.M., Scherpbier, A.J.J., Teunissen, P.W. and Sijtsma, K. (2007) Psychometric properties of an instrument to measure the clinical learning environment Medical education 41(1) p. 92–99

Borton, T. (1970) *Reach, Touch and Teach*. McGraw-Hill, New York.

Boud, D. and Walker, D. (1998) Promoting reflection in professional courses: the challenge of context. *Studies in Higher Education*, 23(2), 191–206.

Botden, S. M. B. I., de Hingh, I. H. J. T. and Jakimowicz, J. J. (2009) Suturing training in augmented reality: gaining proficiency in suturing skills faster. *Surgical Endoscopy* 23 p. 2131–2137

Bowden, J. (2008) Why do nursing students who consider leaving stay on their courses? *Nurse Researcher* 15(3) p. 45–58

Bowers, B., Lauring, C. and Jacobsen, N. (2001) How nurses manage time and work in long-term care. *Journal of Advanced Nursing*, 33(4), 484–491.

Boyd, E. and Fales, A. (1983) Reflective learning: key to learning from experience. *Journal of Humanistic Psychology*, 23(2), 99–117.

Bray, L. and Nettleton, P. (2007) Assessor or mentor? Role confusion in professional education. *Nurse Education Today*. 27 p. 848–855

Bruce, N. (1980) *Teamwork for Preventative Care*. John Wiley and Sons. Research Studies Press, Chichester.

Buchan, J. F. (2011) The chicken or the egg? Investigating the transformational impact of learning technology. *Research in Learning Technology* 19 (2) p. 155–172

Burke, L. and Smith, P. (2000) Developing an audit tool for health promotion learning opportunities in clinical placements. *Nurse Education Today*, 20(6), 475–484.

Burkitt, I., Husband, C., MacKenzie, J. and Tom, A. (2000) *Clinical Judgement and Nurse Education: Nursing Identities and Communities of Practice*. Final Report. University of Bradford and English National Board for Nursing, Midwifery and Health Visiting, London.

Butterworth, T., Carson, J., White, E., Jeacock, J., Clements, A. and Bishop, V. (1997) Clinical Supervision and Mentorship: It's good to talk: An evaluation study in England and Scotland. *University of Manchester*, Department of Nursing and Midwifery, Manchester.

CAIPE (1997) *Interprofessional Education – a definition*. Centre for the Advancement of Interprofessional Education, London.

Callaghan, M. (2003) Nursing morale: what is it like and why? *Journal of Advanced Nursing*, 42(1), 82–89.

Candela, L., Dalley, K. and Benzel-Lindley, J. (2006) A case for learning-centered curricula. *Journal of Nursing Education*, 45(2), 59–66.

Care Quality Commission (2012) [Online] available at http://www.cqc.org.uk/public/about-us

Carper, B. (1978) Fundamental ways of knowing in nursing. *Advances in Nursing Science*, 1(1), 13–23.

Carr, S. M. (2005) Knowing nursing – The challenge of articulating knowing in practice. *Nurse Education in Practice*. 5 p. 333–339

Carr, J., Heggarty, H., Carr, M., Fulwood, D., Goodwin, C., Walker, W. and Whittingham, K. (2010) Reflect for success: recommendations for mentors managing failing students. *British Journal of Community Nursing* 15 (12) p. 594–596.

Carr, H. and Gidman, J. (2012) Juggling the dual role of practitioner and educator: practice teachers' perceptions. *Community Practitioner*. 85 (2) p. 23–26

Casey, D. C. and Clark, L. (2011) Roles and responsibilities of the student nurse mentor: an update. *British Journal of Nursing* 20 (15) p. 933–937

Cassidy, S. (2009) Subjectivity and the valid assessment of pre-registration student nurse clinical learning outcomes: Implications for mentors. *Nurse Education Today*. 29 p. 33–39

Castro, B., Eshleman, J. and Shearer, R. (1999) Using humor to reduce stress and improve relationships. *Seminars for Nurse Managers*, 7(2), 90–92.

Chan, D. (2002) Development of the Clinical Learning Environment Inventory: using the theoretical framework of learning environment studies to assess nursing students' perceptions of the hospital as a learning environment. *Journal of Nursing education.* 41(2) p. 69–75

Channell, W. (2002) Helping students to learn in the clinical environment. *Nursing Times*, 98(39), 34–35.

Chesser-Smyth, P. (2005) The lived experiences of general student nurses on their first clinical placement: a phenomenological study. *Nurse Education in Practice*, 5(6), 320–327.

Cleland, J. A. Knight, L. V. Rees, C. E.Tracey, S. and Bond, C. M. (2008) Is it me or is it them? Factors that influence the passing of underperforming students. *Medical Education* 42 p. 800–809

Coffield, F., Moseley, D., Hall, E. and Ecclestone, K. (2004) *Learning Styles and Pedagogy in Post-16 Learning: A systematic and critical review.* Learning Skills Research Council, London.

Cole, M., John-Steiner, S., Scribner, E. and Souberman, E. (eds) (1978) L. S. *Vygotsky Mind in Society: The development of higher psychological processes.* Harvard University Press, Cambridge, MA.

Collier, J. (2010) Wiki technology in the classroom: building collaboration skills. *Journal of Nursing Education. P.*718

Connexions (2003) *Learning and Young People.* Department for Education and Skills, Sheffield, p.12.

Connor, M. (2004) The practical discourse in philosophy and nursing: an exploration of linkages and shifts in the evolution of praxis. *Nursing Philosophy*, 5(1), 54–66.

Commission on Improving Dignity in Care for Older People (2012) Delivering Dignity [Online] available at **http://www.nhsconfed.org/Publications/ Documents/Delivering_Dignity_final_report**150612. pdf

Cope, P., Cuthbertson, P. and Stoddart, B. (2000) Situated learning in the practice placement. *Journal of Advanced Nursing*, 31(4), 850–856.

Covey, S.R. (2004a) *The 7 habits of highly effective people.* Simon & Schuster. London

Covey, S. R. (2004b) *The 8th Habit.* Simon & Schuster. London

Cowan, J. (1998) *On Becoming an Innovative University Teacher: Reflection in action.* Society for Research into Higher Education and Open University Press, Buckingham.

Cox, J.L., Holden, J.M. and Sagovsky, R. (1987) Detection of postnatal depression: development of the Edinburgh Postnatal Depression Scale. *British Journal of Psychiatry*, **150**, 782–786.

Crawford, M. and Kiger, A. (1998) Development through self-assessment strategies used during clinical nursing placements. *Journal of Advanced Nursing*, 27(1), 157–164.

Crooks, D., Carpio, B., Brown, B., Black, M., O'Mara, L. and Noesgaard, C. (2005) Development of professional confidence by post diploma baccalaureate nursing students. *Nurse Education in Practice*, 5(6), 360–367.

Crotty, M. (1993) Clinical role activities of nurse teachers in Project 2000 programmes. *Journal of Advanced Nursing*, 18, 460–464.

Cushen, N. and Wigens, L. (2000) A staff support mechanism: the transformational partnership. *British Journal of Nursing*, 19(16), 1074–1078.

Darling, L. (1984). What do nurses want in a mentor? *Journal of Nursing Administration*, 14(10), 42–44.

Davey *et al.* (2009) Predictors of nurse absenteeism in hospitals: a systematic review.*Journal of Nursing Management.* 17 p. 312–330

Davies, C. (1995) *Gender and the Professional Predicament in Nursing.* Open University Press, Buckingham.

DeFillippi, R. (2001) Introduction: Project-based learning, reflective practices and learning outcomes. *Management Learning*, 32(1), 5–10.

Department of Health (1997) *Education and Training Plan Guidance.* HMSO, London.

Department of Health (1999) *Making a Difference: Strengthening the nursing, midwifery and health visiting contribution to health and health care.* HMSO, London.

Department of Health (2000a) *Making a Difference in Primary Care: the challenge for nurses, midwives and health visitors.* Case Studies from NHS Regional Conferences. HMSO, London.

Department of Health (2000b) *The NHS Plan – A plan for investment.* A plan for reform. HMSO, London.

Department of Health (2001)'*Working Together – Learning Together*' *A framework for Lifelong Learning.* Department of Health, Crown Publishers London

Department of Health (2004) The NHS Knowledge and Skills Framework (NHSKSF) and Development Review Process. *Department of Health*, Crown Publishers, London.

Department of Health (2008) *A High Quality Workforce.* Department of Health, London.

Department of Health (2010a) *Preceptorship Framework for newly registered nurses, midwives and allied health professionals*. Department of Health, Crown Publishers London.

Department of Health (2010b) Simplified KSF. [Online] available at http://www.nhsemployers.org/payandcontracts/agendaforchange/ksf/simplified-ksf/pages/simplifiedksf.aspx

Department of Health (2010c) *Equity and Excellence: Liberating the NHS* Department of Health, London

Department of Health (2010d) QIPP. [Online] available at www.dh.gov.uk/health/catcgory/policy-areas/nhs/quality/

Department of Health (2011) *Delivering Efficiency savings in the NHS* National Audit Office. London

Department of Health (2012a) *The NHS Constitution for England*. Department of Health, Crown Publishers London

Department of Health (2012b) Briefing notes: issues highlighted by the 2011 NHS staff survey in England. [Online] Availaible at www.nhsstaffsurveys.com (Survey documents/ 2011 results)

de Shazer, S. (1985) *Keys to Solution in Brief Therapy*. New York, NY: Norton.

Dewey, J. (1938) *Experience and Education*. Collier, New York.

Dix, G., Phillips J, and Braide, M. (2012) Engaging staff with intentional rounding. Nursing Times; 108: 3, 14–16.

Dolan, G. (2003) Assessing student nurse clinical competency: will we ever get it right? *Journal of Clinical Nursing*. 12 p. 132–141

Dowswell, T., Hewison, J. and Hinds, M. (1998) Motivational forces affecting participation in post-registration degree courses and effects on home and work life: a qualitative study. *Journal of Advanced Nursing*, 28(6), 1326–1333.

Dreyfus, H. and Dreyfus, S. (1979) *What Computers Can't Do – The limits of artificial intelligence*. The Free Press, New York.

Duffy, K. (2004) *Failing Students*. NMC, London.

Dunn, R. (2003) The Dunn and Dunn learning style model and its theoretical cornerstone. In: *Synthesis of the Dunn and Dunn Learning Styles Model Research: Who, what, when, where and so what – the Dunn and Dunn learning styles model and its theoretical cornerstone* (ed. Dunn, R. and Griggs, S.). St John's University, New York, pp. 1–6.

Dunn, S. and Hansford, B. (1997) Undergraduate nursing students' perceptions of their clinical learning environment. *Journal of Advanced Nursing*, 25(6), 1299–1306.

East Somerset NHS Trust (2000) *Clinical Supervision: Theoretical and practical approaches to the supervision of clinical practice*. East Somerset NHS Trust, Yeovil, Somerset.

Ebright, P., Urden Patterson, E. and Chalko, B. (2004) Themes surrounding novice nurse near-miss and adverse-event situations. *Journal of Nursing Administration*, 34(11), 531–538.

Edmond, C. (2001) A new paradigm for practice education. *Nurse Education Today*, 21(4), 251–259.

Edwards, D., Burnard, P., Hannigan, B., Cooper, L., Adams, J., Juggessur, T., Fothergil, A. and Coyle, D. (2006) Clinical Supervision and burnout: the influence of clinical supervision for community mental health nurses. *Journal of Clinical Nursing* 15(8) p. 1007–1015

Edwards, A. (2012) *New Technology and Education*. Continuum. London.

Elcock, K. and Sookhoo, D. (2007) Research: Evaluating a new role to support mentors in practice (2007) *Nursing Times* 103(49) p. 30–31

Elkan, R. and Robinson, J. (1993) Project 2000: the gap between theory and practice. *Nurse Education Today*, 13(4), 295–298.

Endacott, R., Gray, M., Jasper, M., McMullan, M., Miller, C., Scholes, J. and Webb, C. (2004) Using portfolios in the assessment of learning and competence: the impact of four models. *Nurse Education in Practice*, 4(4), 250–257.

Engestrom, Y. (1994) *Training for Change: New approach to instruction and learning in working life*. International Labour Office, Geneva.

English, F. (1975) The three-cornered contract. *Transactional Analysis*, 5(4), 383–384.

English National Board (1994) *Creating Lifelong Learners: Partnership for care*. London, ENB.

Eraut, M. (1994) *Developing Professional Knowledge and Competence* (4th edn., 1999) Falmer Press, Lewes.

Eraut, M. (1998) Concepts of competence. *Journal of Interprofessional Care* 12 (2) p. 127–139

Eraut, M. (2000a) *The dangers in managing with an inadequate view of knowledge*. A paper presented to the Third International Conference of Sociocultural Psychology – Turning Knowledge Management Upside Down. July, Brazil.

Eraut, M. (2000b) Non-formal learning and tacit knowledge in professional work. *British Journal of Educational Psychology*, 70(1), 113–136.

Eraut, M., Alderton, J., Cole, G. and Senker, P. (1998) Learning from other people at work. In: *Learning at Work* (ed. Coffield, F.). The Policy Press, Bristol.

Farrand, P., McMullan, M., Jowett, R. and Humphreys, A. (2006) Implementing competency recommendations into pre-registration nursing curricula effects upon levels of confidence in clinical skills *Nurse Education Today* 26(2) p. 97–103

Faugier, J. and Butterworth, T. (1992) *Clinical Supervision and Mentorship in Nursing*. Chapman and Hall, London.

Feldman, D. (1999). Toxic mentors or toxic protégés? A critical re-examination of dysfunctional mentoring. *Human Resource Management Review*, 9(3), 247–278.

Field, D. (2004) Moving from novice to expert – the value of learning in clinical practice: a literature review. *Nurse Education Today*, 24(7), 560–565.

Finnerty, G., Graham, L., Magnusson, C. and Pope, R. (2006) Empowering midwife mentors with adequate training and support. British Journal of Midwifery. 14 (4) p. 187–190

Fish, D. and Coles, C. (eds.) (1998) *Developing Professional Judgement in Health Care: Learning through the critical appreciation of practice*. Butterworth Heinemann, Oxford.

Fisher, M., Walsh, A. and Crouch, S. (2005) *Uncovering Skills for Practice*. Nelson Thornes, Cheltenham.

Flagler, S., Lopez-Powers, S. and Spitzer, A. (1988) Clinical teaching is more than evaluation alone! *Journal of Nurse Education*, 27(8), 342–348.

Flanagan, J. (1954) The critical incident technique. *Psychological Bulletin*, 51(4), 327–358.

Fordham, A. J. (2005) Using a competency based approach in nurse education.*Nursing Standard*. 19(31) p. 41–48

Foret Giddens, J., Shucster, G. and Roehrig, N. (2010) Early students outcomes associated with a virtual community for learning. *Journal of Nursing Education*. 49(6) p. 355–358

Foucault, M. (1972) *The Archaeology of Knowledge*. Routledge, London.

Fowler, J., Fenton, G. and Riley, J. (2007) Using solution-focused techniques in clinical supervision. *Nursing Times*. 103 (22) p. 30–31

Fowler, J. (2007) Reflective writing. Thinking and writing at Masters level: a reflective passage. *British Journal of Nursing* 16 (14) p. 887–890

Freeth, D. and Reeves, S. (2004) Learning to work together: using presage, process, and product (3P) model to highlight decisions and possibilities. *Journal of Interprofesssional Care*, 18(1), 43–56.

Gagné, R. (1985) The Conditions of Learning and the Theory of Instruction. *Holt*, Reinhart and Wilson, New York.

Gaines, C., Jenkins, S. and Ashe, W. (2005) Empowering nursing faculty and students for community service. *Journal of Nursing Education*, 44(11), 522–525.

Gee, J. (2004) *Situated Language and Learning: A critique of traditional schooling*. Routledge, London.

Gerrish, K. (2000) Still fumbling along? A comparative study of the newly qualified nurse's perception of the transition from student to qualified nurse. *Journal of Advanced Nursing*, 32(2), 473–480.

George, E., Iveson, C. and Ratner, H. (1999) Problem to Solution: Brief Therapy with Individuals and Families London: B.T. Press

Gibbs, G. (1988) *Learning by Doing: A guide to teaching and learning methods*. Oxford Further Education Unit, Oxford.

Giddens, J., Fogg, L. and Carlson-Sabell, L. (2010) Learning and engagement with a virtual community by undergraduate nursing students. *Nursing Outlook* 58 (5) p. 261–267

Glasper, A. (2010a) The care quality commission criteria for assessing NHS Trusts. British Journal of Nursing 19 (5) p. 280–281

Glasper, A. (2010b) Additional options for achieving sign-off mentor criteria. *British Journal of Nursing* 19(10) p. 658–659.

Goleman, D. (1995) *Emotional Intelligence*. Bantam Books, New York.

Good, J., Howland, K. and Thackray, L. (2008) Problem-based learning spanning real and virtual words: a case study in Second Life, *ALT-J Research in Learning Technology* 16(3) p. 163–172

Goodman, J. (1989) Reflection and teacher education: a case study and theoretical analysis. *Interchange*, 15(3), 9–26.

Gopee, N. (2002) Human and social capital as facilitators of lifelong learning initiated through informal facilitators of learning through work based contacts with other health care professionals. *Nurse Education Today*, 22(8), 608–616.

Gopee, N. (2011) *Mentoring and Supervision in Healthcare* 2nd ed. Sage. London

Gopee, N. (2008) Assessing student nurses' clinical skills: The ethical competence of mentors. *International Journal of Therapy and Rehabilitation*. 15 (9) p. 401–407

Gough, P. (2001) Changing culture and deprofessionalisation. *Nursing Management*, 7(9), 8–9.

Gover, S. and Heathershaw, R. J. R (2011) 'Focus on assessment' as part of unpublished project work exploring Practice Assessment.

Grant, A. (2000) Clinical supervision and organisational power: a qualitative study. *Health and Learning Disabilities Care*, 3(12), 398–401.

Greenhalgh, T. and Worrall, J. (1997) From EBM to CSM: the evolution of context sensitive medicine. *Journal of Evaluation in Clinical Practice*, 3(2), 105–108.

Gurling, J. (2011) Link mentorship: improving support for pre-registration students and mentors. *British Journal of Community Nursing* 16 (9) p. 435–440

Hallsten *et al.* (2011) Job burnout and job wornout as risk factors for long-term sickness absence, *Work*. 38 p. 181–192

Hall, V. and Hart, A. (2004) The use of imagination in professional education to enable learning about disadvantaged clients. *Learning in Health and Social Care*, 3(4), 190–202.

Hammick, M. (2000) Interprofessional education: evidence from the past to guide the future. *Medical Teacher*, 22(5), 472–478.

Hand, H. (2006) Promoting effective teaching and learning in the clinical setting.

Handy, C, (1999) Understanding Organizations . Penguin. London

Harries, C. (2011) Concerns over practice education ratios. Community Practitioner. 84(9) p. 16–18

Harrison, R., Reeve, F., Hanson, A. and Clarke, J. (2002) (eds.) *Supporting Lifelong Learning*. Vol. 1. Perspectives on Learning. Routledge Falmer, London.

Hart, G. and Rotem, A. (1995) The clinical learning environment: nurse perceptions of professional development in clinical practice. *Nurse Education Today*, 15(1), 3–10.

Harvey, G., Loftus-Hills, A., Rycroft-Malone, J., Titchen, A., Kitson, A., McCormack, B. and Seers, K. (2002) Getting evidence into practice: the role and function of facilitation. *Journal of Advanced Nursing*, 37(6), 577–588.

Harvey-Lloyd, J. (2008) Unpublished 'Workplace Coaching' module, adapted from Whitworth L, Kimsey-House, H. and Davies, S. (1998). Co-active coaching. Black Publishing. Califormia and NMC (2008) Standards to support learning and assessment in practice. NMC London.

Hatton, N. and Smith, D. (1995) Reflection in teacher education – towards definition and implementation. *Teaching and Teacher Education*, 11(1), 33–49.

Hawkins, P. and Shohet, R. (1989) *Supervision in the Helping Professions: An individual, group and organizational approach*. Open University Press, Milton Keynes.

Haydock, D., Mannix, J. and Gidman J. (2011) CPTs' perceptions of their role satisfaction and levels of professional burnout, 84 (5) p. 19–23

Health Professions Council (2011) *Your guide to our standards for continuing professional development*. HPC. London.

Heitlinger, A. (1999) Nurses and nursing: a comparative perspective. *Journal of Interprofessional Care*, 13(2),

Henderson, A., Winch, S. and Heel, A. (2006) Partner, learn, progress: a conceptual model for continuous clinical education. *Nurse Education Today*, 26(2), 104–109.

Heron, J. (1989) Six Category Intervention Analysis. *Human potential resource group*, University of Surrey, Guildford.

Hewinson, A. (1999) Nurses' power in interaction with patients. *Journal of Advanced Nursing*, 21(1), 75–82.

Hewison, A., Badger, F. and Swani, T. (2011) Leading end-of-life care: an action learning set approach in nursing homes. *International Journal of Palliative Nursing*. 17(3) p. 135–141

Higher Education National Academy (2006) *National Professional Standards Framework for Teaching and Supporting Learning in Higher Education*. HENA, London.

Hochschild, A. (1983) *The Managed Heart: commercialisation of human feeling*. University of California Press, Berkeley.

Hogan, M., Kapralos, B., Cristancho, S., Finney, K. and Dubrowski, A. (2011) Bringing community health nursing education to life with serious games. International Journal of Nursing Scholarship. 8(1) art. 8

Honey, P. and Mumford, A. (1992) *The Manual of Learning Styles*. Peter Honey Publications, Maidenhead.

Houle, C. (1961) *The Inquiring Mind: A study of the adult who continues to learn*. University of Wisconsin Press, *Madison. Updated edition (1988) Research Center for Continuing Professional and Higher Education*, University of Oklahoma, McCarter Hall.

Howell, W. and Fleishman, E. (1982) (eds.) *Human Performance and Productivity*. Vol. 2. Information Processing and Decision Making. Erlbaum, Hillsdale, NJ.

Hughes, E. (2005) Nurses' perceptions of continuing professional development. *Nursing Standard* 19(43) p. 41–49

Hughes, A.J. and Fraser, D.M. (2011) Sink or Swim: The experience of newly qualified midwives in England. *Midwifery* 27(3) p. 382–386

Hyatt, S. A., Brown, L. and Lipp, A. (2008) Supporting mentors as assessors of clinical practice.Nursing Standard. 22(25) p. 35–41

Illeris, K. (2007) *How we learn*. Routledge. Abingdon

Ioannides, A. (1999) The nurse teacher's clinical role now and in the future. *Nurse Education Today*, **19**(3), 207–214.

Jacobs-Kramer, M. and Chinn, P. (1988) Perspectives on knowing: a model of nursing. *Scholarly Inquiry for Nursing Practice*, **2**(2), 129–139.

James, N. (1992) Care = Organisation + physical labour + emotional labour. *Sociology of Health and Illness*, **14**(5), 488–509.

Jarvis, P. (1995) *Adult and Continuing Education: Theory and practice*. Routledge, London.

Jarvis, P. and Gibson, S. (1997) *The Teacher Practitioner in Nursing, Midwifery and Health Visiting*, 2nd edn. Stanley Thornes Publishers, Cheltenham.

Jasper, M. (1996) The portfolio workbook as a strategy for student centred learning. In: *Closing the Theory–Practice Gap* (ed. Rolfe, G.). Butterworth Heinemann, Oxford.

Jasper, M. (2003) *Beginning Reflective Practice. Foundations in Nursing and Health Care*. Nelson Thornes, Cheltenham.

Jasper, M. (2013) *Foundations in Nursing and Health Care. Beginning Reflective Practice*. (2nd Edition) Cengage.

Jasper, M. (2013) *Beginning Reflective Practice*. (2nd Edition) Cengage Learning EMEA

Jasper, M. and Fulton, J. (2005) Marking criteria for assessing practice-based portfolios at masters' level. *Nurse Education Today*, **25**(5), 377–389.

Jervis, A. and Tilki, M. (2011) Why are nurse mentors failing to fail student nurses who do meet clnical performance standards? British Journal of Nursing **20**(9) p. 582–587

JISC (2012) Crossing the Threshold: moving e-portfolios into the mainstream [Online] available from http://www.jisc.ac.uk/whatwedo/programmes/elearning/eportfolios/crossing.aspx

JISC (2012) Learning in a digital age [Online] available from http://www.jisc.ac.uk/whatwedo/programmes/elearning/digilifelong.aspx

Johns, C. (2000) *Becoming a Reflective Practitioner*. Blackwell Science, Oxford.

Johns, C. (2006) Engaging reflection in practice – A narrative approach. Blackwell Science. Oxford.

Johns, C. (2009)*Becoming a Reflective Practitioner 3rd ed*. Wiley Blackwell. Chichester

Johns, C. and Freshwater, D. (1998) *Transforming Nursing Through Reflective Practice*. Blackwell, Oxford.

Johnson, L., Adams, S.Cummins, M. (2012*) The NMC Horizon Report: 2012 Higher Education Edition*. Austin Texas: The New Media Consortium

Johnson, D. and Johnson, R. (1992) *Advanced Cooperative Learning*. Interaction, MN.

Jowett, R. and McMullan, M. (2007) Learning in practice – practice educator role. *Nurse Education in Practice* 7 p. 266–271

Kadushin, A. (1992) *Supervision in Social Work, 3rd. edn*. Columbia University Press, New York.

Kilcullen, N.M. (2007) The impact of mentorship on clinical learning.Nursing Forum **42**(2) pp. 95–104

Kings College London (2012) Intentional rounding: what is the evidence? Policy plus evidence, issues and opinions in healthcare. 35 April 2012.

Kirkpatrick, D. (1975) Techniques for Evaluating Training Programmes. *American Society for Training and Development*, Alexandria, VA.

Knowles, M. (1986) *Using Learning Contracts*. Jossey-Bass, San Francisco, CA.

Knowles, M. (1990) *The Adult Learner – A neglected species*. Gulf Publishing, Houston.

Koh, L. (2002) Practice-based teaching and nurse education. *Nursing Standard*, **16**(19), 38–42.

Kolb, D. (1984a) *Experiential Learning: Experience as a source of learning development*. Prentice Hall, Englewood Cliffs, NJ.

Kolb, D. (1984b) *Experiential Learning as the Science of Learning and Development*. Prentice Hall, Englewood Cliffs, NJ.

Kramer, M. (1974) *Reality Shock: Why nurses leave nursing*. Mosby, St Louis, MO.

Kristiansen, M. and Bloch-Poulsen, J. (2004) Self-referentiality as a power mechanism: towards dialogic action research. *Action Research*, **2**(4), 371–388.

Kyrkjebø, J. and Hage, I. (2005) What we know and what they do: nursing students' experiences of improvement knowledge in clinical practice. *Nurse Education Today*, **25**, 167–175.

Lauder, W., Reynolds, W. and Angus, N. (1999) Transfer of knowledge and skills: some implications for nursing and nurse education. *Nurse Education Today*, **19**(6), 480–487.

Lauder, W., Sharkey, S. and Booth, S. (2003) A case study of transfer of learning in a family health nursing course for students in remote and rural areas. *Nurse Education in Practice*, **4**(1), 39–44.

Lave, J. and Wenger, E. (1991) *Situated Learning – Legitimate Peripheral Participation*. Cambridge University Press, Cambridge.

Lawler, L. (1991) *Behind the Screens: Nursing, somology, and the problem of the body*. Churchill Livingstone, Melbourne.

LeMay, A. (1999) Knowledge for dissemination and implementation. In: *Nursing Research: Dissemination and implementation* (ed. Mulhall, A. and LeMay, A). Churchill Livingstone, Edinburgh.

Levett-Jones, T. (2005) Continuing education for nurses: a necessity or a nicety? *Journal of Continuing Education in Nursing*, 36(5), 229–233.

Levett-Jones, T. and Lathlean, J. (2009) The ascent to competence conceptual framework: an outcome of a study of belongingness *Journal of Clinical Nursing* 18 p. 2870–2879

Levett-Jones, T, Lathlean, J, Higgins, I. McMillan, M. (2009) Staff-student relationships and their impact on nursing students' belongingness and learning. *Journal of Advanced Nursing*. 65(2), 316–324.

Lewin, K. (1942) Field theory and learning. In: *Field Theory in Social Science: Selected theoretical papers* (1951) (ed. Cartwright, D.). Social Science Paperbacks, London.

Lines, H and Ricketts, B. (1994) Learning to achieve transformation in health. In: *Towards the Learning Company: Concepts and practices* (ed. Burgoyne, J., Pedler, M. and Boydell, T.). McGraw-Hill Book Company, London, Chapter 13, 158–168.

Little, V. (1999) The meaning of learning in critical care nursing: a hermeneutic study. *Journal of Advanced Nursing*, 30(3), 697–703.

Luhanga, F., Yonge, O. and Myrick, F. (2008) Failure to assign failing grades: Issues with grading the unsafe student. International Journal of Nursing Education Scholarship. 5(1) art. 8

Lymn, J. and Bowskill, D. (2010) Learning on the move *Nursing Standard* 24(31) p. 61

Macdonald, R. and Savin-Baden, M. (2004) *Assessment in Problem-Based Learning*. LTSN Generic Centre Assessment Series, No.7. LTSN Generic Centre, York.

Mackereth, P. (1989) An investigation of the developmental influences on nurse's motivation for their continuing education. *Journal of Advanced Nursing*, 14(9), 776–778.

Maeve, M. (1998) Weaving a fabric of moral meaning: how nurses live with suffering and death. *Journal of Advanced Nursing*, 27(6), 1136–1142.

Magnussen, L. (2008) 'Applying principles of significant learning in the e-learning environment' *Journal of Nursing Education*. 47 (2) pp. 82–85

Malik M. and McGowan B. (2007) Issues in practice based learning in nursing in the United Kingdom and the Republic of Ireland: Results from a multi professional scoping exercise. *Nurse Education Today* 27 p. 52–59

Manley, K. and McCormack, B. (1997) *Exploring Expert Practice (NUM65U)*. Royal College of Nursing, London.

Manley, K., Hardy, S., Titchen, A., Garbett, R. and McCormack, B. (2005) *Changing Patients' Worlds Through Nursing Practice Expertise*. A Royal College of Nursing Research Report, 1998–2004. RCN, London.

Marinker, M. (1974) Medical education and human values. *Journal of the Royal College of General Practitioners*, 24(144), 445–62.

Marton, F. and Saljo, R. (1984) Approaches to learning. In: *The Experience of Learning* (ed. Marton, F., Hounsell, D. and Entwhistle, N.). Scottish Academic Press, Edinburgh.

Maslow, A. (1954) *Motivation and Personality*. Harper, New York.

Maslow, A. (1970) *Motivation and Personality*. Harper and Row, New York.

Maudsley, G. and Strivens, J. (2000) Promoting professional knowledge, experiential learning and critical thinking for medical students. *Medical Education*, 34(7), 535–544.

McAllister, M. (2003) Doing practice differently: solution-focused nursing. *Journal of Advanced Nursing*, 41(6), 528–535.

McArthur, G. S. and Burns, I. (2008) An evaluation, at the 1-year stage, of a 3 year project to introduce practice education facilitators to NHS Tayside and Fife. *Nurse Education in Practice*. 8 p. 149–155

McCormack, B., Kitson, A., Harvey, G., Rycroft-Malone J., Titchen, A. and Seers, K. (2002) Getting evidence into practice: the meaning of 'context'. *Journal of Advanced Nursing*, 38(1), 94–104.

McGarry, J. and Thorn, N. (2004) How users and carers view their involvement in nurse education. *Nursing Times*, 100(18), 36–39.

McGonigle, D. and Eggers, R. (2001) Editorial: Introduction – A student in the not too distant future. [Online] *Journals of Nursing Informatics (OJNI) 15 (2)* available at http://ojni.org/issues/?p=620

McGowan, B. (2006) *Who do they think they are? Undergraduate perceptions of the definition of supernumery status and how it works in practice Journal of Clinical Nursing* 15 p. 1099–1105

McMullan, M. (2005) Competence and its assessment - a review of the literature. British Journal of Podiatry. 8 (2) p. 49–52

McMullan, M., Endacott, R., Gray, M., Jasper, M., Miller, C., Scholes, J. and Webb, C. (2003) Portfolios and assessment of competence: a review of the literature. *Journal of Advanced Nursing*, 41(3), 283–294.

Mead, D. (2011) Views of nurse mentors about their role. *Nursing Management* 18 (6) p. 18–23

Melia, K. (1987) *Learning and Working: The occupational socialization of nurses*. London, Tavistock.

Memletics (2004) Memletics Learning styles inventory [online] Available at http://www.crs.sk/storage/memletics-learning-styles-inventory.pdf

Menzies, I. (1960) *The Functioning of Social Systems as a Defence Against Anxiety: A report on a study of the nursing service of a general hospital.* Tavistock, London.

Miers, M. (2002) Nurse education in higher education: understanding cultural barriers to progress. *Nurse Education Today*, 22(3), 212–219.

Mikkelsen Kyrkjebø, J. and Hage, I. (2005) What we know and what they do: nursing students' experiences of improvement knowledge in clinical practice. *Nurse Education Today*, 25(3), 167–175.

Mohammed, M. (2004) Using statistical process control to improve the quality of health care. *Quality and Safety in Health Care*, 13(4), 243–245.

Moon, J. (1999) *Reflection in Learning and Professional Development: Theory and Practice.* Kogan Page, London.

Mooney, M. (2007a) Professional socialisation : the key to survival as a newly qualified nurse. *International Journal of Nursing Practice* 13 p. 75–80

Mooney, M. (2007b) Newly qualified Irish nurses interpretation of their preparation and experinces of registration. *Journals of Clinical Nursing.* p. 1610–1617

Moores, A. and Parks M. (2010) Twelve tips for introducing E-portfolios with undergraduate students *Medical Teacher* 32 p. 46–49

Morgan, C., Dunn, L., Parry, S. and O'Reilly, M. (2004) *The student assessement handbook: New directions in traditional and Online assessment.* Routledge. London

Morton-Cooper, A. and Palmer, A. (1993) *Mentoring and Preceptorship.* Blackwell Science, Oxford.

Moseley, L. G. and Davies, M. (2007) What do mentors find difficult? *Journal of Clinical Nursing.* P. 1627–1634

Moseley, L., Mead, D. and Moran, L. (2004) An empirically derived clinical placement evaluation tool: a 3-country study. *Nurse Education Today*, 24(5), 350–356.

Mulhall, A. (2002) Nursing research and nursing practice: an exploration of two different cultures. *Intensive and Critical Care Nursing*, 18(1), 48–55.

Myall, M. Levett-Jones, T. and Lathlean, J. (2008) Mentorship in contemporary practice: the experiences of nursing students and practice mentors. *Journal of Clinical Nursing.* p. 1834–1842

Myers, I. and McCaulley, M. (1998) *Manual: A guide to the development and use of the Myers-Briggs Type Indicator.* Consulting Psychologists Press, Palo Alto, CA.

Myrick, F. and Yonge, O. (2001) Creating a climate for critical thinking in the preceptorship experience. *Nurse Education Today*, 21(6), 461–467.

NHS Employers (2012) NHS terms and conditions of service handbook. Amendment number 27. [Online] Accessed via www.nhsemployers.org/PayAndContracts/AgendaForChange

NHS Institute for Innovation and Improvement (2009) Inspiring change in the NHS: introducing five frames. [Online] available at www.changemodel.nhs.uk/dl/cv_content/13772

Nicol, M. and Freeth, D. (1998) Assessment of clinical skills: a new approach to an old problem. *Nurse Education Today*, 18(8), 601–609.

Northouse, P. G. (2009) *Leadership: Theory and Practice 5th ed.* Sage. London

Nursing and Midwifery Council (2004b) *Midwives Rules and Standards.* NMC, London.

Nursing and Midwifery Council (2006) *Standard to support learning and assessment in practice.* NMC, London.

Nursing and Midwifery Council (2008) *Standard to Support Learning and Assessment in Practice* NMC London.

Nursing and Midwifery Council (2010a) *NMC circular 05/2010 Sign-off Mentor criteria.* NMC London.

Nursing and Midwifery Council (2010b) Standards for Pre-registration Nurse Education. NMC London

Nursing and Midwifery Council (2011a) *The Prep handbook.* [Online] available at http://www.nmc-uk.org/Documents/Standards/NMC_Prep-handbook_2011.pdf

Nursing and Midwifery Council (2011b) *Guidance on Professional conduct for nursing and midwifery students* NMC London

Oakshott, M. (1962) *Rationalism in Politics and Other Essays.* Methuen and Co., London.

Ohlen, J. and Segesten, K. (1998) The professional identity of the nurse: concept analysis and development. *Journal of Advanced Nursing*, 28(4), 720–727.

Ohrling, K. and Hallberg, I. (2001a) Nurses' lived experience of being a preceptor. *Journal of Professional Nursing*, 16(4), 228–239.

Ohrling, K. and Hallberg, I. (2001b) The meaning of preceptorship: nurses' lived experience of being a preceptor. *Journal of Advanced Nursing*, 33(4), 530–554.

Oliver, R. and Endersby, C. (2000) *Teaching and Assessing Nurses: A handbook for preceptors.* Bailliere Tindall, London.

Omansky, G. L. (2010) Staff nurses' experiences as preceptors and mentors: an integrative review. *Journal of Nursing Management.* **18** p. 697–703.

Orland-Barak, L. and Wilhelem, D. (2005) Novices in clinical practice settings: student nurses' stories of learning the practice of nursing. *Journal of Advanced Nursing*, **21**(1), 75–82.

Palmer, A., Burns, S. and Bulam, C. (1994) *Reflective Practice in Nursing: The growth of the professional practitioner.* Blackwell Science, Oxford.

Palmer S., Harmer Cox, A., Callister, L., Johnsen, V. and Matsumura, G. (2005) Nursing education and service collaboration: making a difference in the clinical learning environment. *Journal of Continuing Education in Nursing*, **36**(6), 271–276.

Papastavrou, E., Lambrinou, E., Tsangari, H., Saarikoski, M. and Leino –Kilpi, H. (2010) Student nurses experience of learning in the clinical environment *Nurse Education Practice* 10, 3, 176–182

Papp, I., Markkanen, M. and von Bonsdorff, M. (2003) Clinical environment as a learning environment: student nurses' perceptions concerning clinical learning experiences. *Nurse Education Today*, **23**(4), 262–268.

Pardoe, S. (2000) A question of attribution: the interdeterminacy of learning from experience. In: *Student Writing in Higher Education* (ed. Lea, M. and Stierer, B.). SRHE/ Open University Press, Milton Keynes, pp. 123–145.

Parliamentary and Health Service Ombudsman (2011) *Care and compassion? Report of the Health Service Ombudsman on ten investigations into NHS care of older people.* HMSO London.

Parsons, T. (1968) Professions. In: *International Encyclopaedia of the Social Sciences* (ed. Sills, D.). Macmillan, New York, **xii**, pp. 536–547.

Patel, V., Arocha, J. and Kayfman, D. (1999) Medical cognition. In: *Handbook of Applied Cognition* (ed. Durso, F.). Wiley, New York, pp. 663–693.

Pearce, R. (2003) *Profiles and Portfolios of Evidence.* Foundations in Nursing and Health Care. Nelson Thornes, Cheltenham.

Pearcey, P. and Elliott, B. (2004) Student impressions of clinical nursing. *Nurse Education Today*, **24**(5), 382–387.

Perry-Woodford, Z. and Whayman, K. (2005) Education in practice: a colorectal link-nurse programme. *British Journal of Nursing*, **14**(16), 862–866.

Peyton, J. (1998) The learning cycle. In: *Teaching and Learning in Medical Practice* (ed. Peyton, J.). Manticore, Rickmansworth, pp. 13–19.

Pfeil, M. (2003) Assessing the clinical skills performance of nursing students. *Journal of Child Health Care*, 7(3), 191–206.

Phillips, T., Schostak, J. and Tyler, J. (2000a) *Practice and Assessment: An evaluation of the assessment of practice at diploma, degree and postgraduate level in pre and post registration nursing and midwifery education.* English National Board for Nursing, Midwifery and Health Visiting, London.

Phillips, T., Schostak, J. and Tyler, J. (2000b) *Practice and Assessment in Nursing and Midwifery: Doing it for real* (PandA project). English National Board, London.

Piaget, J. (1971) *Biology and Knowledge.* Edinburgh University Press, Edinburgh.

Pirrie, A., Wilson, V., Elsegood, J., Hall, J., Hamilton, S., Harden, R., Lee, D. and Stead, J. (1998) *Evaluating Multidisciplinary Education in Health Care.* Scottish Council for Research Education, Edinburgh.

Playle, P. and Mullarkey, K. (1998) Parallel process in clinical supervision: enhancing learning and providing support. *Nurse Education Today*, 18(7), 558–566.

Polanyi, M. (1951) *The Logic of Liberty.* Routledge and Kegan Paul, London.

Price, B. (2004) Encouraging reflection and critical thinking in practice. Nursing Standard, 18(47), 46–52.

Price, B. (2007) Practice-based assessment: strategies for mentors. *Nursing Standard.* 21 (36) p. 49–56

Price, S.L (2008) Becoming a nurse: a meta-study of early professional socialization and career choice in nursing. *Journal of Advanced Nursing 65 (1) p. 11–19*

Priest, H. (1999) Novice and expert perceptions of psychological care and the development of psychological caregiving abilities. *Nurse Education Today*, **19**(7), 556–563.

Proctor, B. (1987) Supervision: A co-operative exercise in accountability. In: *Enabling and Ensuring: Supervision in practice* (ed. Marken, M. and Payne, M.). National Youth Bureau, Leicester.

Quality Assurance Agency for Higher Education (2001) *Code of Practice for the Assurance of Academic Quality and Standards in Higher Education.* Section 9: Placement Learning. QAAHE, Gloucester.

Quinn, F.M. and Hughes, S.J. (2007) *Quinn's principles and practice of nurse education* (5th edn). Nelson Thornes, Cheltenham.

Ramsden, P. (1992) *Learning to Teach in Higher Education.* Routledge, London.

Randle, J. (2003) Changes in self-esteem during a 3-year pre-registration Diploma in Higher Education (Nursing) programme. *Journal of Clinical Nursing*, **12**(1), 142–143.

Richardson, B. (1999) Professional development: 2 Professional knowledge and situated learning in the workplace. *Physiotherapy*, **85**(9), 467–474.

Robinson, A., Murrell, T., Hickey, G., Clinton, M. and Tingle A. (2003) *A Tale of Two Courses: Comparing careers and competencies of nurses prepared via a three-year degree and three-year diploma courses*. Kings College, Nursing Research Unit, London.

Rogers, C. (1967) The interpersonal relationships in the facilitation of learning. In: *Humanizing Education* (ed. Leeper, R). Association for Supervision and Curriculum Development, Alexandria VA.

Rogoff, B. (1990) *Apprenticeship in Thinking*. Oxford University Press, New York and Oxford.

Rolfe, G. (1993) Closing the theory-practice gap: a model of nursing praxis. *Journal of Clinical Nursing*, **2**(3), 173–177.

Rolfe, G. (2006) Nursing praxis and the science of the unique. *Nursing Science Quarterly*, **19**(1), 39–43.

Royal College of Nursing (2002a) *Helping Students Get the Best from Their Practice Placements: a Royal College of Nursing toolkit*. RCN, London.

Royal College of Nursing (2003) *The Future Nurse*. RCN Policy Unit, London.

Royal College of Nursing (2004) *The Future Nurse: The future for nurse education: a discussion paper*. RCN, London.

Royal College of Nursing (2010) *Dyslexia, dyspraxia and dyscalculia: a toolkit for nursing staff*. RCN, London.

Rutowski, K. (2007) Failure to fail: assessing nursing students' competence during practice placements. *Nursing Standard* 22 (13) p. 35–40

Ryan, J. (2003) Continuous professional development along the continuum of lifelong learning. *Nurse Education Today*, **23**(7), 498–508.

Sarup, M. (1996) *Identity, Culture and the Postmodern World*. Edinburgh University Press, Edinburgh.

Saunders, L. (1998) Managing delegation: a field study of a systematic approach to delegation in out-patient physiotherapy. *Physiotherapy*, **84**(11), 547–555.

Savin-Baden, M. (2000) *Problem-based Learning in Higher Education: Untold stories*. Open University Press, Buckingham.

Scanlon, J. and Chernomas, W. (1997) Developing the reflective teacher. *Journal of Advanced Nursing*, **25**(6), 1138–1143.

Scheffer, B. and Rubenfeld, M. (2000). A consensus statement on critical thinking in nursing. *Journal of Nursing Education*, **39**(8), 352–362.

Scholes, J., Webb, C., Gray, M., Endacott, R., Miller, C., Jasper, M. and McMullan, M. (2004). Making portfolios work in practice. *Journal of Advanced Nursing*, **46**(6), 595–603.

Schön, D. (1983) *The Reflective Practitioner: How professionals think in action*. Basic Books, New York.

Schostak, J. Davis, M. Hanson, J. Schostak, J. Brown, T. Driscoll, P. Starke, I. Jenkins, N. (2010) 'Effectiveness of continuing professional development' project: A summary of findings *Medical Teacher* 32 p. 586–592

Schuler, R. and Jackson, S. (1986) Managing Stress through PHRM practices: An uncertainty interpretation. In: *Research in Personnel and Human Resource Management*, Vol. 4. (ed. Rowland, R. and Ferris, G.). JAI Press, Greenwich, CT, pp. 183–224.

Selwyn, N. (2011) *Education and Technology* Contiuum London

Senge, P. (2006) *The Fifth Discipline*. Random house. London

Sharples, K. (2008) No obstacle to success *Nursing Standard*. 22 (51) p. 61

Simons, H. and Parry-Crooke, G. (2001) *We All Thrive on Praise: The Certificate in Teaching for Medicine and Dentistry*. Independent External Evaluation. Kent, Surrey and Sussex Deanery.

Skiba, D. J. (2005) E-portfolios, webfolio and e-identity *Nursing Education Perspectives* 26 (4) p. 246–247

Skinner, B. (1953) *Science and Human Behavior*. The Free Press, New York.

Sloan, G. (2005) Clinical supervision: beginning the supervisory relationship. *British Journal of Nursing*, **14**(17), 918–923.

Sloan, G. and Watson, H. (2001) John Heron's six-category intervention analysis: towards understanding interpersonal relations and progressing the delivery of clinical supervision for mental health nursing in the United Kingdom. *Journal of Advanced Nursing*, **26**(2), 206–214.

Smith, J. and Topping, A. (2001) Unpacking the 'value added' impact of continuing professional education: a multi-method case study approach. *Nurse Education Today*, **21**(5), 341–349.

Smith, P. (1992) *The Emotional Labour of Nursing: How nurses care*. Macmillan, London.

Spouse, J. (1998) Learning to Nurse through legitimate peripheral participation. *Nurse Education Today* 18(5) p. 345–351

Spouse, J. (2003) *Professional Learning in Nursing*. Blackwell, Oxford.

Staib, S. (2003). Teaching and measuring critical thinking. *Journal of Nursing Education*, **42**(11), 498–508.

Steinaker, N. and Bell, R. (1979) *The Experiential Taxonomy: A new approach to teaching and learning*. Academic Press, New York.

Stephenson, J. (1992) Capability and quality in higher education. In: *Quality in Learning: A capability approach in higher education* (ed. Stephenson, J. and Weil, S.). Kogan Page, London.

Stephenson, K., Peloquin, S., Richmond, S., Hinman, M. and Christiansen, C. (2002) Changing educational paradigms to prepare health professionals for the 21st century. *Education for Health*, **15**(1), 37–49.

Stevens, K. and Ledbetter, C. (2000) Basics of evidence based practice. Part 1: The nature of evidence. *Seminars in Perioperative Nursing*, **9**(3), 91–97.

Stoltenberg, C. D. and Delworth, U. (1987) *Supervising Counsellors and Therapists*. Jossey-Bass, San Francisco, CA.

Stordeur, S., D'Hoore, W. and Vandenberghe, C. (2001) Leadership, organizational stress, and emotional exhaustion among hospital nursing staff. *Journal of Advanced Nursing*, **35**(4), 533–542.

Strachan, R., Liyanage, L., Casselden, B. and Penlington, R. (2011) Effectiveness of technology to support work based learning: the stakeholders' perspective. ALT-C Conference Proceedings p. 134–144

Stuart, C. (2007) Assessment, Supervision and Support in Clinical Practice 2nd ed. Churchill Livingstone. London

Suikkala, A. and. Leino-Kilpi, H. (2005) Nursing student–patient relationship: experiences of students and patients. *Nurse Education Today*, **25**(5), 344–354.

Taylor, J., Irvine, F., Bradbury-Jones, C. and McKenna, H. (2010) On the precipice of great things: The current state of UK Nurse Education. *Nurse Education Today*. 30 p. 239–244

Taylor, T. and Nichol, D. (2011) Supporting practice-based learning with video-mediated technologies: an overview. *International Journal of Therapy and Rehabilitation*. 18 (9) p. 513–518

Tennant, M. (2005) *Psychology and Adult Learning*, 3rd edn. Routledge, London.

Theodosius, C. (2008) *Emotional Labour in Health Care. The unmanaged heart of nursing*. Routledge. London.

Thompson, C., McCaughan, D., Cullum, N., Shelden, T., Mulhall, A. and Thompson, D. (2001) Research information in nurses' clinical decision-making: What is useful? *Journal of Advanced Nursing*, **36**(3), 376–388.

Thorndike, E. (1913) The psychology of learning. *Educational Psychology* 2, Teachers' College Columbia University, New York.

Thorpe, K. (2004) Reflective learning journals: from concept to practice. *Reflective Practice*, **5**(3), 1–18.

Titchen, A. (2000) Professional craft knowledge in patient-centred nursing and facilitation of its development. Unpublished PhD Thesis. University of Oxford, Oxford.

Titmus, C. (1999) Concepts and practices of education and adult education: obstacles to lifelong education and lifelong learning. *International Journal of Lifelong Education*, **18**(3), 343–354.

Tiwari, A. and Tang, C. (2003) From process to outcome: the effect of portfolio assessment on student learning. *Nurse Education Today*, **23**(4), 269–277.

Towle, A., Bainbridge, L., Godolphin, W., Katz, A., Kline, C., Lown, B., Madularu, I., Solomon, P. and Thistlewaite J. (2010) Active patient involvement in the education of health professionals. *Medical Education*, **44**,1, 56–74

Traxler, J. (2009) 'Current state of mobile learning' in Ally M. (ed) *Mobile Learning Transforming the delivery of education and training* AU Press Edmonton AB.

Traxler, J. (2010) Students and mobile devices. *ALT-J Research in Learning Technology* **18**(2) p. 149–160

Tryssenar, J. and Perkins, J. (2001) From student to therapist: exploring the first year of practice. *American Journal of Occupational Therapy*, **55**(1), 19–27.

Tucker, B., Jones, S., Mandy, A., and Gupta, R. (2006) Physiotherapy students' sources of stress, perceived course difficulty, and paid employment: Comparison between Western Australia and United Kingdom. *Physiotherapy theory and Practice*. 22 (6) p. 317–328

Tuckman, B. and Jensen, M. (1977). Stages of small group development revisited. *Group and Organization Studies*, **2**(4), 419–427.

Tye, C. and Ross, F. (2000) Blurring boundaries: professional perspectives of the ENP role in a major accident and emergency department. *Journal of Advanced Nursing*, **31**(5), 1089–1096.

United Kingdom Central Council for Nursing Midwifery and Health Visiting (1996) *Position Statement on Clinical Supervision for Nursing and Health Visiting*. UKCC London.

United Kingdom Central Council for Nursing, Midwifery and Health Visiting and Department of Health (1999) *Fitness for Practice*. UKCC, London.

Usher, R. and Soloman, N. (1999) Experiential learning and the shaping of subjectivity in the workplace. *Studies in the Education of Adults*, 31(2), 155–163.

Wagner, F. (1957). Supervision of psychotherapy. *American Journal of Psychotherapy*, 11(4), 759–768.

Wallace, B. (2003) Practical issues of student assessment. *Nursing Standard*, 17(31), 33–36.

Walsh, D. (2010) *The Nurse Mentor's Handbook*. McGraw-Hill. Maidenhead.

Walsh, M. and Crumbie, A. (20110 Initial evaluation of Stilwell: a multimedia virtual community. *Nurse Education in Practice*. 11 p. 136–140

Walsh, M. and Wigens, L. (2003) *Introduction to Research*. Nelson Thornes, Cheltenham.

Ward, K. and Hartley, J. (2006) Using a virtual learning environment to address one problem with problem based learning. *Nurse Education in Practice*. 6 p. 185–191

Wanless, D. (2004) *Securing Good Health for the Whole Population*. HM Treasury, London.

Waskett, C. (2006) Solution-focused supervision. Healthcare Counselling and Psychotherapy. In therapy Today 17, 2, 40-42.

Watson, R., Stimpson, A., Topping, A. and Dorock, D. (2002) Clinical competence assessment in nursing: a systematic review of the literature. Journal of Advanced Nursing. 39 (5) p. 421–431

Weidman, J., Twale., D. and Stein, E. (2001) Socialisation of graduate and professional students in higher education. *ASHE-ERIC Higher Education Report*, 28(3), Wiley Interscience, San Francisco.

Wellard, S. J., Bethune, E. and Heggen, K. (2007) Assessment of learning in contemporary nurse education: Do we need standardised examination for nurse registration? Nurse Education Today. 27 p. 68–72

Wenger, E. (1998) *Communities of Practice: Learning, meaning and identity*. Cambridge University Press, Cambridge.

Wenger, E. McDermott, R. and Snyder, W. (2002) *Cultivating Communities of Practice*. Harvard Business School Press, Boston.

Whitsed, N. (2005) Learning and teaching *Health Information and Libraries Journal* 22 p. 74–77

Wigens, L. (1997) The conflict between 'new nursing' and 'scientific management' as perceived by surgical nurses. *Journal of Advanced Nursing*, 25(6), 1116–1122.

Wigens, L. (1999) The impact of an English National Board breast care course [ENB NO9] on registered nurses' interprofessional collaboration. Conference Presentation: Breakthrough Breast Cancer Conference, London.

Wigens, L. (2004) A case study of registered (care of the adult) nurses' management of individual caring in multiple demand settings, and the influence on this of situated learning. Unpublished PhD thesis. Norwich, University of East Anglia.

Wigens, L. (2005) Care in the multidisciplinary team. In: *Principles of Caring* (ed. McGee, P.). Nelson Thornes, Cheltenham.

Wigens, L. and Westwood, S. (2000) Issues surrounding educational preparation for intensive care nursing in the 21st century. *Intensive and Critical Care Nursing*, 16(4), 221–227.

Wildman, S., Weale, A., Rodney, C. and Pritchard, J. (1999) The impact of higher education for post-registration nurses on their subsequent clinical practice: an exploration of students' views. *Journal of Advanced Nursing*, 29(1), 246–253.

Wilkes, Z. (2006) The student mentor relationship: a review of the literature. *Nursing Standard*. 20 (37) p. 42–47.

Williams, A. and Sibbald, B. (1999) Changing roles and identities in primary health care: exploring a culture of uncertainty. *Journal of Advanced Nursing*, 29(3), 737–745.

Williams, P. (1998) Using theories of professional knowledge and reflective practice to influence educational change. *Medical Teacher*, 20(1), 28–34.

Williamson, G. and Dodds, S. (1999) The effectiveness of a group approach to clinical supervision in reducing stress: a review of the literature. *Journal of Clinical Nursing*, 8(4), 338–344.

Williamson, W. Callaghan, L. Whittlesea, E. and Heath, V. (2010) Improving student support using Placement Development teams: staff and student perceptions. *Journal of Clinical Nursing*. 20 p. 828–836.

Wilson, G. and Randall, M. (2012) The implementation and evaluation of a new learning space: a pilot study. *Research in Learning Technology*. 20

Wilson-Barnett, J., Butterworth, T., White, E., Twinn, S., Davies, S. and Riley, L. (1995) Clinical support and the Project 2000 nursing student: factors influencing this process. *Journal of Advanced Nursing*, 21(6), 1152–

Wolff, A. and Rideout, E. (2001). The faculty role in problem-based learning. In: *Transforming Nursing Education through Problem-based Learning* (ed. Rideout, E). *Jones and Bartlett*, Sudbury, MA.

Wood, I. (1998) The ENB 199: an exploration of its effects on A & E nurses' practice. *Accident and Emergency Nursing*, 6(4), 219–225.

Wood, G. Harben-Obasuyi, J. and Richardson, M. (2011) Clinical Practice Facilitator: A new role to support mentors and students. *British Journal of Midwifery* 19 (8) p. 526–528

Woodcock, J. (2009) Supporting students who may fail. *Emergency Nurse* 16(9), 18–21.

Worral, K. (2007) Orientation to student placements: needs and benefits. *Paediatric Nurse* 19 (1) p. 31–33

Young, B. (2009) Shining a light on care *Nursing Management* 15 (10) p. 14–16

INDEX